蜡型堆塑教程
WAXING
FOR
DENTAL
STUDENTS

（埃及）罗维达·阿布达拉（Rowida Abdalla） 编著

赵 今 林 静 主译

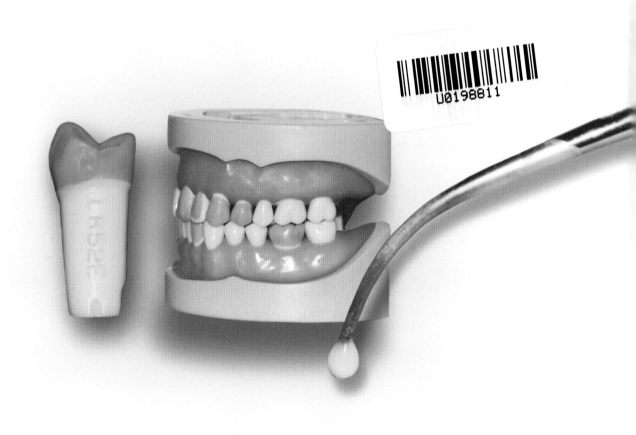

北方联合出版传媒（集团）股份有限公司

辽宁科学技术出版社

沈 阳

主译简介
Translators

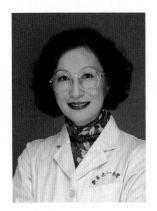

赵 今

新疆医科大学口腔医学院教授，博士研究生。新疆医科大学第一附属医院（附属口腔医院）院长，国际牙医师学院（ICD）中国区院士，享受国务院特殊津贴专家。先后主持国家级和省部级科研项目10项，发表论文200余篇，其中SCI收录20余篇。参编第八轮全国高等学校口腔医学专业五年制本科教育部、国家卫生计生委"十三五"规划教材《牙体牙髓病学》《口腔医学》《口腔科学》等国家级教材6部，主编省部级论著2部，副主编论著2部。担任《现代口腔医学杂志》副主编，《华西口腔医学杂志》《口腔疾病防治》《新疆医科大学学报》编委。先后获得新疆维吾尔自治区科技进步奖二等奖3项；新疆医学科技奖二等奖2项。主持教育教学改革项目6项。荣获霍英东教育基金会教育教学二等奖，省部级教学成果奖三等奖，校级教学成果奖二等奖。兼任中华口腔医学会理事会常务理事、中华口腔医学会牙体牙髓病学专业委员会常务委员，中国医院协会口腔医院分会常务委员，新疆口腔医学会会长，教育部高等学校口腔医学专业教学指导委员会委员，全国高等学校口腔医学专业教材评审委员会委员。先后获得新疆维吾尔自治区有突出贡献优秀专家、自治区教学名师、"天山英才"专家、最美科技工作者等称号。

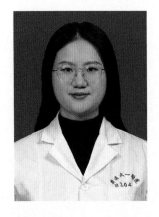

林 静

新疆医科大学口腔医学院副主任医师。先后主持省部级科研项目3项，发表论文10余篇。参编《口腔门诊常见疾病PBL案例教学》教师版和学生版。先后获得新疆维吾尔自治区科技进步2项；新疆医学科技奖2项。兼任中华口腔医学会牙体牙髓病学专业委员会青年委员、中华口腔医学会口腔医学教育专业委员会委员、新疆口腔医学会牙体牙髓病学专业委员会常务委员。

译者名单

赵 今　林 静　吴泽钰　姬晓炜　张洋洋　夏雨凝

以上译者均来自新疆医科大学第一附属医院（附属口腔医院）

前言
Preface

本书是为牙科学校一年级的学生提供的蜡型堆塑学习指南。本书提供了一种循序渐进的方法，学习部分和全冠蜡型堆塑，参照解剖学和形态学标准，并以模型上的对侧同名牙为参照。书中提供了1~2个各种牙齿堆塑的案例。可以按照同样的步骤堆塑不同牙齿的蜡型。本书对蜡型堆塑的形态学进行了详细的解释，并给出了最终蜡型堆塑的形态学目标。但本书并不是形态学的教科书。

而且，本书中堆塑的蜡型没有形成咬合。通过对切/殆面形态进行精准的堆塑，以获得合适的尺寸和轮廓；但是，并未呈现咬合接触的内容。另外，也有其他图书以供学习在咬合状态下蜡型堆塑的技巧。

按照本书所呈现的内容顺序学习是至关重要的，因为这一顺序使学生能够逐渐提升他们的技能水平。学生可从简单的入门练习开始，熟悉器械握持和蜡型堆塑。而后是进行切牙、尖牙、前磨牙和磨牙的全冠蜡型堆塑。学生通过使用本书最后一章中的评价标准来评价他们的作品。

This book serves as a manual of waxing teeth for students in their first year of dental school. The manual provides a step-by-step approach to partial and full-crown wax-ups that are anatomically and morphologically correct and match the contralateral tooth on the dentoform. This book provides one or two examples of waxing every tooth type. This book can be used for waxing different teeth by following the same steps. The morphology of the teeth waxed in this guide is explained in detail as a reminder of the morphologic goal of the final wax-up. However, this manual is not a textbook on morphology.

Furthermore, the teeth in this manual are not waxed into occlusion. Waxing the occlusal/incisal morphology is done precisely and accurately to proper dimensions and contour; however, achieving occlusal contacts is not a part of this guide. There are several books available for learning techniques of waxing in occlusion.

It is crucial to use this book in the sequence in which it is presented, as this sequence enables students to develop their skills gradually. Students begin with simple introductory exercises to familiarize themselves with holding instruments and handling wax. This is followed by waxing full-crowns of incisors, canines, premolars, and molars. Students should evaluate their work using the evaluation rubric in the last chapter of this book.

中文版前言
Preface

本书是现就职于美国加州大学洛杉矶分校牙科学院的罗维达·阿布达拉教授编写的关于口腔医学实验教学领域的图书，很荣幸能将其翻译成为我国口腔医学实验教学类用书。

本书提供了丰富的实验教学案例和操作指南，是口腔医学实验教学教师们的得力助手，为教师们设计课程和实验教学提供了有力支持。教师们可以根据本书的内容，灵活组织实验教学环节，引导学生逐步掌握蜡型堆塑技巧，将理论知识与实践操作相结合，培养动手能力和临床思维。

学习和掌握蜡型堆塑技巧对于每一位口腔医学生都很重要，蜡型堆塑是口腔解剖生理学、牙体牙髓病学和口腔修复学等学习中的重要环节之一。在牙体缺损修复和修复体制作等临床工作中，熟练的蜡型堆塑是准确还原牙齿形态和结构的基础。本书从基础知识到高级技巧，层层递进，简明扼要地呈现了蜡型堆塑的精髓。学生可以通过系统学习，掌握蜡型堆塑工具的正确使用要点、不同牙位蜡型堆塑的特点与应用，以及实际操作的要领，有助于在日后的临床实践中自信和熟练地运用所学技能，提高治疗质量。

希望本书能够在口腔医学实验教学中发挥积极作用，愿每一位教师和学生都能从中汲取知识，不断进步，提高我国口腔医学教育教学水平。

感谢原著作者贡献的资料，感谢所有参与本书翻译和编辑的工作人员，感谢辽宁科学技术出版社给予的重视和支持，将这本优质的实验教学图书呈现给广大读者。

赵 今

新疆医科大学第一附属医院（附属口腔医院）

目录
Contents

扫一扫即可浏览
参考文献

第1章
Chapter

蜡型堆塑概论
Introduction to Waxing

蜡型堆塑目的

蜡型大部分由技工中心的技工制作，使用失蜡法来制作间接修复体。当计划行前牙修复时，医生可以通过制作蜡型来帮助自己实现最好的治疗效果，同时蜡型也是一种和患者有效沟通的工具。对于学生来说，制作蜡型的主要目的是学习每颗牙齿的形态和解剖结构，这样在行修复治疗时，学生才能把牙齿恢复到正确的形态。

位于牙弓内的每颗牙齿都有5个面。这些面都不是完全平坦的：不同部位和不同类型的牙齿，每个面都有其独特的凹凸形态。在进行牙体修复时应该精确地恢复牙齿的解剖标志，这样才能使其达到良好的美学形态和功能。制作蜡型正是练习如何正确复制牙体形态的绝佳途径。此外，口腔医学生们在制作蜡型的过程中可以熟悉手用器械的使用，增加手指的灵活性及手部操作的稳定性，提高专注度和缩短反应时间。这些技能在要求高精确度操作的牙科中十分重要。

Purpose of Waxing Teeth

Waxing teeth is mainly done by laboratory technicians to fabricate indirect restorations using the lost wax technique. When anterior restorations are planned, waxing can also be done by the dentist to achieve the best possible outcome; it can as well be an effective patient communication tool. For students, the main purpose for waxing teeth is to learn the morphology and anatomy of each individual tooth, so you are able to eventually restore teeth to the correct form.

Each tooth in the dental arch has five surfaces. Those surfaces are not flat: Every surface has convexities and concavities that are unique to its location and tooth type. Anatomical landmarks should be duplicated precisely when teeth are restored so that good esthetics and function can be achieved. Waxing is a great exercise to learn how to duplicate the correct tooth contours. In addition, the process of waxing familiarizes dental students with hand instrumentation techniques and allows them to develop skills such as finger dexterity, hand steadiness, aiming, and reaction time. These skills are essential for the high precision needed in dentistry.

蜡型堆塑器械

- Bunsen喷灯和气管
- 堆塑工具：PKT1、PKT2、蜡刀、PKT3、PKT4（Hollenback雕刻刀）以及盘–爪状雕刻刀（大工作尖和小工作尖）
- 铸造蜡：Renfert GEO Classic铸造–不透明造型蜡（75g）
- 牙科操作练习模型D85SDP–200（Kilgore International），内含28颗牙齿和软质牙龈
- 螺丝刀
- Kilgore模型牙（解剖式）
- Kilgore A21AN–200系列预备牙
  - 唇侧#22 UL29D
  - 切端、唇侧、舌侧#12 UR24
  - 全冠#32 LL21A
  - 全冠#21 UL11C
  - 全冠#23 UL31D
  - 颊侧、𬌗面、近中#24 UL49H
  - 全冠#24 UL42B
  - 全冠#45 LR52E
  - 𬌗面、近中、远中、舌侧#16 UR66C
  - 全冠#36 LL62D
- 尼龙布
- 铅笔
- 超细黑色记号笔
- 防护眼镜

工作台的设置

　　牙科临床和实验室对工作台的组织管理是工作精确性及效率的重要保证。合理规划与使用器械将加快工作和学习的提升进程。操作者需要在一个组织有序、供应良好的工作场所工作（图1-1）。

Waxing Armamentarium

- Bunsen burner and tubing.
- Waxing instruments: PKT1, PKT2, waxing spatula, PKT3, PKT4 (ie, Hollenback carver), and two discoid-cleoid carvers (large and small).
- Casting wax: Renfert GEO Classic mint-opaque modeling wax (75 gm) .
- Dental Typodont Model D85SDP-200 (Kilgore International) with 28 teeth and soft gingiva.
- Screwdriver.
- Kilgore model teeth (anatomical replica).
- Kilgore A21AN-200 Series Prep Teeth.
  - Facial #22 UL29D
  - Incisal labial lingual #12 UR24
  - Full-crown #32 LL21A
  - Full-crown #21 UL11C
  - Full-crown #23 UL31D
  - Facial, occlusal, mesial #24 UL49H
  - Full-crown #24 UL42B
  - Full-crown #45 LR52E
  - Occlusal, mesial, distal, lingual #16 UR66C
  - Full-crown #36 LL62D
- Nylon stockings.
- Pencil.
- Ultrafine-point black marker.
- Eye shields.

Setup of the Work Station

The nature of the precision and efficiency of clinical and laboratory work in dentistry mandates organization of the work area. The use of instrument setups and the availability of needed items will expedite your work and facilitate the learning process. It is expected that you will work from an organized and properly supplied work station (Fig 1-1).

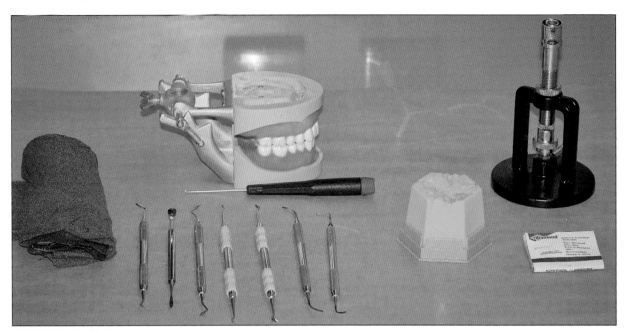

图1-1

制作蜡型所需工具

　　蜡型工具分为堆蜡和雕蜡两种[1-2]（图1-2和图1-3）。

堆蜡工具

　　PKT1用于堆蜡（图1-2a）。工作尖呈弯曲状，一端为圆形，一端为锥形，并且手柄能安全加热。

　　PKT2也用于堆蜡，并且有一个尖的工作尖，可以用于填补牙尖嵴、唇/颊轴和舌轴轮廓以及𬌗面之间空隙或瑕疵（图1-2b）。

　　蜡刀用于最开始堆蜡或后牙堆蜡时加入大量的蜡（图1-2c）。它也可以加热后用来平整较大范围的蜡表面。

Waxing instruments

Waxing instruments are divided into wax-addition and wax-carving categories[1,2] (Figs 1-2 and 1-3).

Wax-addition instruments

PKT1. Used to apply wax (Fig 1-2a). The tips are round, curved, and tapered and the shank can be safely heated.
PKT2. Also used to apply wax and featuring a pointed tip that can be used to fill in voids or discrepancies between the crest of cusp ridges and the facial and lingual axial contours and on the occlusal surface (Fig 1-2b).
Waxing spatula. Used to add a large amount of wax in the initial step of waxing or when waxing posterior teeth (Fig 1-2c). It can also be heated and applied to smooth a large surface.

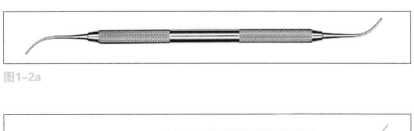

图1-2a

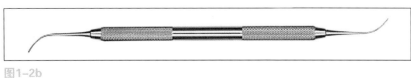

图1-2b

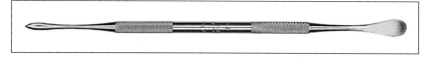

图1-2c

雕蜡工具

　　这些工具是待蜡冷却后用来雕刻蜡型的，不应该被加热。

　　PKT3的特征是带有尖头磨光器，用于完善和加深窝沟形态（图1-3a）。

　　PKT4用于完善外部轮廓和清除边缘多余的蜡（图1-3b），也称为Hollenback雕刻刀。

　　盘–爪状雕刻刀用于雕刻舌窝、三角窝以及唇/颊发育沟（图1-3c）。小工作尖雕刻前牙，大工作尖雕刻后牙。

Wax-carving instruments

These instruments are used to carve the wax after it cools. They are *not* meant to be heated.

PKT3. Features a pointed burnisher and is used to perfect and enhance supplemental and developmental grooves (Fig 1-3a).

PKT4. Used to perfect the external contours and remove the excess wax at the margin (Fig 1-3b). It is also known as a *Hollenback carver*.

Discoid-cleoid carver. Used to carve the lingual and triangular fossae and facial developmental depressions (Fig 1-3c). The small one can be used for anterior teeth and the large one can be used for posterior teeth.

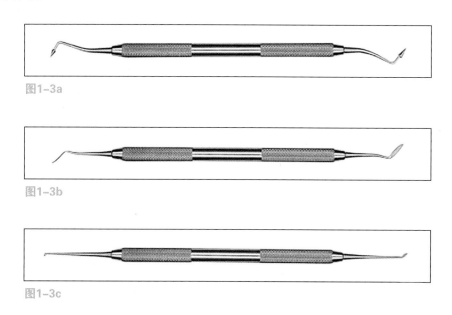

图1-3a

图1-3b

图1-3c

器械握持

　　改良握笔法是在蜡型堆塑和大多数修复过程中使用手用器械时最容易掌握的姿势（图1-4a）。当给牙列模型外堆蜡时，使用非惯用手握持牙，使用惯用手以改良握笔法握持器械，并把无名指放在可摘代模上形成支点保持稳定（图1-4b）。

Holding the Instruments

The modified pen grasp is the easiest when waxing teeth and for using hand instruments in most restorative procedures (Fig 1-4a). When waxing outside the dentoform, you will hold the tooth with your nondominant hand and the instrument with your dominant hand in a modified pen grasp with your ring finger resting on the tooth peg for stability and precision (Fig 1-4b).

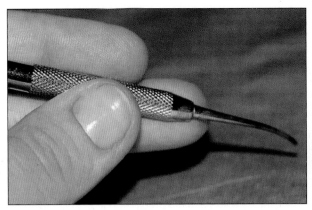

图1-4a

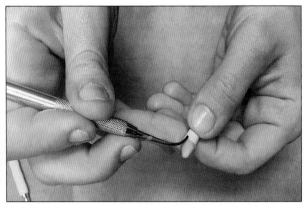

图1-4b

Bunsen喷灯的使用

　　Bunsen喷灯可以分别手动调节燃气和空气的流量。燃气由实验台燃气阀通过橡胶管输送到Bunsen喷灯底部。燃气流量由灯底部的小旋钮调节，转动灯底部的套筒，可以打开或关闭进气孔来调节气流。点燃Bunsen喷灯时，需确保其周围完全清空，实验室中没有易燃溶剂[3]。

Bunsen喷灯使用说明[3]

1. 将气管连接至实验台上的燃气阀处（图1-5a）。
2. 调整Bunsen喷灯底部的气体调节旋钮使燃气流速适中，并旋转灯底部的套筒，使空气流动几乎完全停止（图1-5b）。
3. 划一根火柴或使用打火机，将火源靠近灯的一侧，但不要完全接触它（图1-5c），同时打开实验台燃气阀（图1-5d）。使用火柴或打火机在Bunsen喷灯顶部附近产生火花。灯点燃后发出的火焰为蓝色，火焰越蓝，表明温度越高。这些是通过允许更多的空气进入来实现的。调整燃气和空气流量，使火焰达到想要的大小，并使火焰有明显的蓝色外焰和内焰（图1-6）。
4. 要熄灭Bunsen喷灯时，只需关闭实验台上的燃气阀。

Bunsen Burner Use

A Bunsen burner is designed so that gas and airflow can be regulated separately and manually. Gas is delivered from the lab bench gas valve to the base of the Bunsen burner via a rubber tube. Gas flow is regulated with the small knob at the base of the burner, and rotating the sleeve at the base of the burner to open or close the air-inlet holes regulates airflow. When lighting a Bunsen burner, make sure the area around the burner is completely clear and that no flammable solvents are in use in the laboratory.[3]

Instructions for lighting the Bunsen burner[3]

1. Connect the tubing to the gas valve on the lab bench (Fig 1-5a).
2. Adjust the gas regulator knob on the bottom of the Bunsen burner for a moderate flow of gas, and rotate the sleeve at the base of the burner so that airflow is almost completely closed off (Fig 1-5b).
3. Strike a match or use a lighter and hold it close to the side of the burner, but not quite touching it (Fig 1-5c), while you turn on the bench gas valve (Fig 1-5d). Use the match/lighter to produce sparks near the top of the Bunsen burner. The lit flame will be blue and the bluer the flame, the hotter it will be. This is achieved by allowing more air into the mixture. Adjust the gas and airflow to produce a flame of the desired size that has two distinct blue regions (Fig 1-6). The hottest part of the flame is the tip of the inner dark blue cone.
4. To extinguish a Bunsen burner, simply turn off the gas at the bench valve.

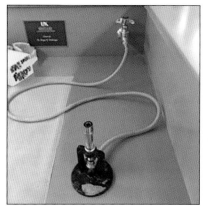

图1–5a

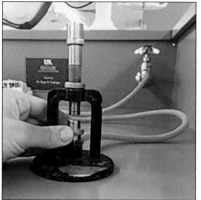

图1–5b

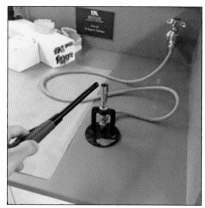

图1–5c

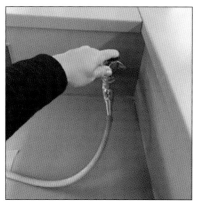

图1–5d

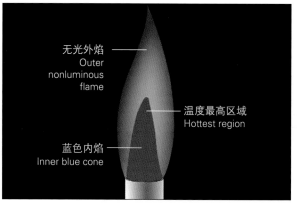

图1–6

无光外焰
Outer nonluminous flame

温度最高区域
Hottest region

蓝色内焰
Inner blue cone

堆蜡技术

堆蜡技术是指一种通过有序及连续地添加蜡来形成所需解剖结构的过程。将取蜡器的工作尖置于Bunsen喷灯火焰中加热（图1–7a），再与蜡接触（图1–7b），然后将工作尖再次放入火焰中快速加热[1]。一颗蜡珠会从工作尖的顶端流出（图1–7c）。如果蜡过热，它会流下并形成很大的一个平面。用蜡覆盖可摘代模表面或颊/舌侧是堆蜡的最初步骤。为了使蜡珠形成牙尖状凸起或嵴状凸起，蜡应该保持足够热度（图1–7d~f），但温度不能过高。这需要在取蜡后等待1~2秒，再让工具接触牙面。

Wax-Addition Technique

The wax-addition technique is the process used to develop a wax pattern through an organized, sequential addition of wax to shape the individual components of the desired anatomical form. Wax is added by heating the shank of the wax-addition instrument in the Bunsen flame (Fig 1-7a), touching it to the wax (Fig 1-7b), and quickly reheating the shank in the flame.[1] A bead of wax will flow away from the tip of the instrument (Fig 1-7c). If the wax is too warm, it will pool and cover a large surface. This is done in the initial waxing steps when the tooth peg surface is being covered with wax or whenever the facial and lingual surfaces are waxed. To form more confined beads for building cusps or ridges, the wax should be warm enough but not too warm (Figs 1-7d to 1-7f). This requires waiting a second or two before letting the instrument touch the tooth surface.

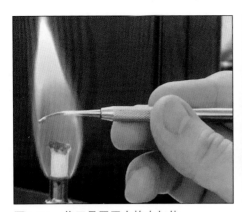

图1-7a 将工具置于火焰中加热
Heating the instrument in the flame.

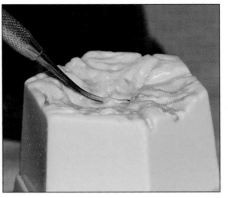

图1-7b 使用加热后的工具接触蜡
Touch the hot instrument to the wax.

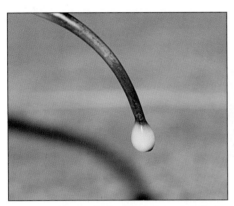

图1-7c 蜡从工作尖顶端流出，形成蜡珠
Wax flows off the tip and forms a bead.

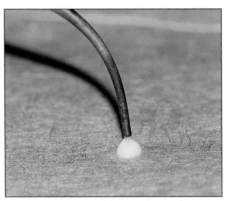

图1-7d 将工作尖靠近表面，堆入蜡珠
Touch the instrument tip to the surface to add wax beads.

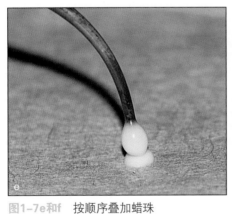

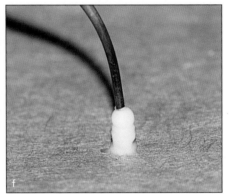

图1-7e和f 按顺序叠加蜡珠
Sequential addition of wax beads.

堆塑全冠的标准化方法

Standardized Approach to Waxing Full-Crowns

每颗牙齿都有其独特的解剖特征，当制作蜡型或修复体时应该体现出这些特征。然而，个体差异是存在的，而且不是每颗牙齿都能达到最好

Each tooth has well-known anatomical features that should be duplicated when the tooth is waxed or restored. However, individual variations do exist, and what is ideal may not give the best esthetic or functional

的美学效果或功能恢复。因此，制作蜡型和修复体的目标是与对侧同名牙外形匹配，与邻牙及对颌牙协调。邻面接触区例外，即使修复体没有邻牙，也应在制作时恢复到正确的接触关系及位置。

- 遵循一系列逻辑步骤并参考解剖学
  - 可摘代模
  - 邻牙
  - 对侧同名牙
  - 对颌牙
- 单纯追求美学形态是十分困难的

解剖形态参考

- 对侧同名牙线角
- 对侧同名牙点角
- 邻牙和对侧同名牙外形高点
- 邻牙和对侧同名牙邻接
- 对侧同名牙楔状隙
- 邻牙和对侧同名牙唇面及舌面
- 邻牙和对侧同名牙边缘嵴
- 邻牙和对侧同名牙舌窝
- 邻牙和对侧同名牙舌轴嵴
- 邻牙和对侧同名牙切缘
- 邻牙和对侧同名牙牙尖
- 邻牙中央窝
- 对侧同名牙𬌗面形态

轮廓成形规则

1. **唇/颊面外形高点**位于所有牙齿解剖牙冠的颈1/3[4]（图1-8）。
2. **舌面外形高点**，前牙位于解剖牙冠的颈1/3，后牙位于解剖牙冠的中1/3（图1-8）[4]。
3. 唇/颊面和舌面外形高点突出唇/颊侧及舌侧颈缘线以外0.5mm内[5]（图1-9）。

results in every dentition. Therefore, the goal during waxing and restoring teeth is to match the contralateral tooth contours and achieve harmony with the adjacent and opposing teeth. One exception is the proximal contact, which should be waxed/restored to achieve proper closure and position, even if the contralateral proximal contact on your dentoform is open.

- Follow a logical series of steps using anatomical references that are present on:
  - Tooth peg
  - Adjacent teeth
  - Contralateral tooth
  - Opposing teeth
- A purely artistic approach is very difficult.

Anatomical references

- Contralateral line angles.
- Contralateral point angles.
- Adjacent and contralateral heights of contour.
- Adjacent and contralateral proximal contact areas.
- Contralateral embrasures.
- Adjacent and contralateral labial and lingual surfaces.
- Adjacent and contralateral marginal ridges.
- Adjacent and contralateral lingual fossae.
- Adjacent and contralateral cingulae.
- Adjacent and contralateral incisal edges.
- Adjacent and contralateral cusps.
- Adjacent central grooves.
- Contralateral occlusal morphology.

Rules for Developing Contours

1. The **facial height of contour** is located in the cervical third of the anatomical crowns of all teeth[4] (Fig 1-8).
2. The **lingual height of contour** is located in the cervical third of anatomical crowns of anterior teeth and the middle third of the anatomical crowns of posterior teeth[4] (see Fig 1-8).
3. The facial and lingual heights of contours do not extend more than 0.5 mm beyond the cervical line faciolingually[5] (Fig 1-9).

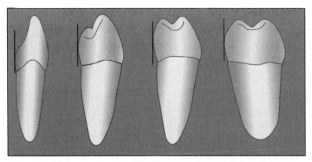

图1-8

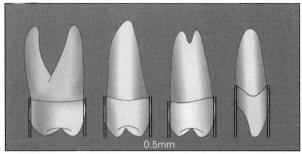

0.5mm

图1-9

4. **上颌牙齿的唇/颊面**在颈1/3外形高点与殆面或切端之间有轻微的凸起，不呈一条直线[5]（图1-10）。

5. **下颌后牙的颊面**在颈部外形高点和殆面之间呈现明显的凸起（图1-11）。要建立美观和有助于发音的颊面轮廓，应参考邻牙外形[5]。

4. The **facial surfaces of maxillary teeth** present a very slight convexity, rather than a straight profile, between the facial height of contour at the cervical third and the occlusal or incisal surface[5] (Fig 1-10).

5. The **facial surfaces of mandibular posterior teeth** present a pronounced convexity between the cervical height of contour and the occlusal surface (Fig 1-11). To establish facial contours that are esthetic and phonetic, they should be influenced by those of adjacent teeth.[5]

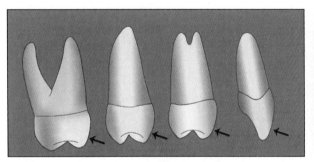

图1-10

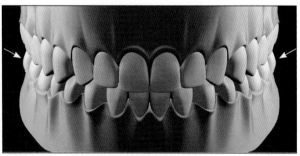

图1-11

6. 离中线越远，**邻面接触区**越接近牙龈（图1-12）。中切牙的近中、远中接触区位于切1/3处，侧切牙近中接触区位于切1/3处，尖牙远中接触区位于中1/3处。后牙邻面接触区位于殆1/3和中1/3交界处[6-7]。

6. **Interproximal contacts** are situated progressively closer to the gingiva the more distal they are located from the midline (Fig 1-12). Interproximal contacts occur at the incisal thirds for central incisors, at the junction of the incisal and middle thirds at the mesial of the lateral incisors, and at the center of the middle third at the distal of the canine. The proximal contacts of posterior teeth occur at the middle thirds or the junction of the occlusal and middle thirds.[6,7]

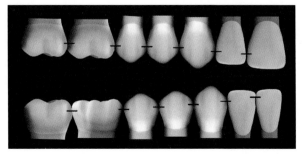

图1-12

7. **邻面接触区**位于唇舌径/颊舌径中央偏颊侧，导致舌楔状隙比颊楔状隙大[4-6]（图1-13）。

7. Faciolingually, the **proximal contact areas** are facial to the faciolingual center of the tooth, resulting in lingual embrasures that are larger than the buccal embrasures[4-6] (Fig 1-13).

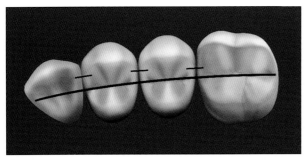

图1-13a

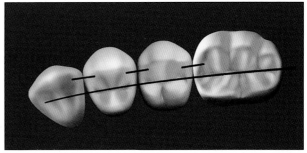

图1-13b

8. 每颗牙齿邻面接触区与釉牙骨质界之间，邻面接触区颈2/3的各个方向（唇颊径和𬌗颈向）的形态都是比较平整的[5]（图1-14）。

- 规则7和规则8中的例外是，相对于上颌第一磨牙的远中接触区，其邻面接触区位于牙冠颊舌向和𬌗颈向的中心。相应地，该牙远中面外形是突出的[5]（图1-15）

8. The cervical two-thirds of the proximal surface of each tooth is flat in both directions (faciolingually and occlusocervically) between the proximal contact and the cementoenamel junction[5] (Fig 1-14).

- The exception to rules 7 and 8 is that for the distal surface of the maxillary first molar, the proximal contact is at the center of the crown buccolingually and occlusocervically. Correspondingly, the distal surface of that tooth is convex[5] (Fig 1-15).

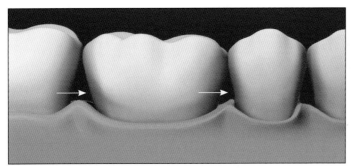

图1-14a

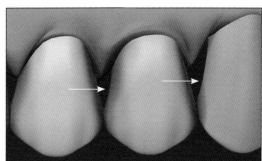

图1-14b

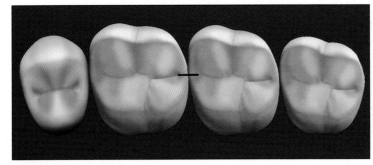

图1-15a

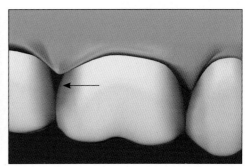

图1-15b

9. **边缘嵴**：呈圆形，隆起的嵴形成前牙舌侧近远中边缘和后牙𬌗面近远中边缘（图1-16a）。所有相邻的边缘嵴应在同一高度，以防食物嵌塞和滞留。所有边缘嵴都从颊侧向舌侧聚合。因此，所有牙齿的唇/颊侧都比舌侧宽，舌楔状隙都比颊楔状隙大[5]（图1-16b）。

9. **Marginal ridges** are rounded, elevated crests forming the mesial and distal margins of the lingual surface of anterior teeth and the occlusal surface of posterior teeth (Fig 1-16a). All adjacent marginal ridges should be at the same height to prevent food impaction and retention. All marginal ridges converge from the buccal toward the lingual. Therefore, the facial half of any tooth is wider than the lingual half, and the lingual embrasure is always larger than the buccal embrasure[5] (Fig 1-16b).

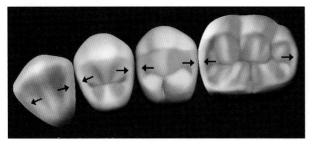

图1-16a

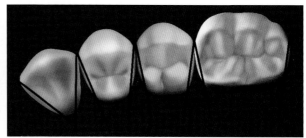

图1-16b

10. **楔状隙**：两颗邻牙邻接之间形成的V字形空间（图1-17）。V字形空间的最窄部分在邻接区。面向唇/颊侧的间隙形成唇/颊楔状隙，面向舌侧的间隙形成舌楔状隙，面向切面/𬌗面的间隙变宽形成切/𬌗楔状隙，颈部间隙变宽形成龈/颈邻间隙。可以从切面观或𬌗面观来看颊楔状隙和舌楔状隙，从唇/颊面观和舌面观来看颈邻间隙和切/𬌗楔状隙。所有的蜡型或修复体的楔状隙大小、位置都应与对侧同名牙一致[6]。

10. An **embrasure** is a V-shaped space adjacent to the contact area of two adjacent teeth (Fig 1-17). The narrowest part of the V-shaped space is at the contact area. The space widens facially to form the facial embrasure, lingually to form the lingual embrasure, occlusally to form the incisal/occlusal embrasure, and cervically to form the gingival/cervical embrasure. The facial and lingual embrasures can be viewed from an incisal/occlusal view, and the cervical and occlusal/incisal embrasures can be viewed from both buccal and lingual views. All embrasures of the wax-up or a dental restoration should be identical in size and location to those of the contralateral tooth.[6]

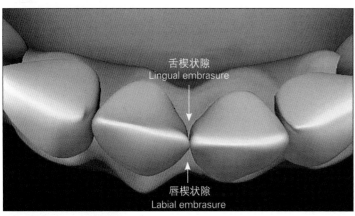

图1-17a

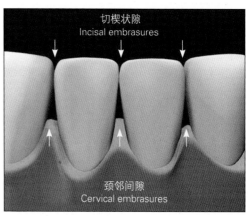

图1-17b

11. **线角**：两个相邻牙面相交处形成一线——邻面或切/殆面与唇/颊面或舌面相交[5]（图1–18）。线角在邻接和釉牙骨质界之间较平直，除了上颌磨牙的舌侧线角和上颌前牙唇侧线角呈弧形，远唇线角比近唇线角更圆突。前牙的唇侧线角决定了其唇面外形[1]。线角的外形应该建立在美学和形态学的基础上，形态与对侧同名牙一致。

11. **Line angles** occur at the junction between two surfaces—a proximal or incisal/occlusal surface with a facial or lingual surface[5] (Fig 1-18). Line angles are generally straight between the proximal contact and the cementoenamel junction, except the lingual line angles of maxillary molars and the labial line angles of maxillary anterior teeth are usually rounded, the distolabial being more convex than the mesiolabial line angle. The labial line angles of anterior teeth determine the appearance of their labial surface.[1] Line angles should be established esthetically and morphologically to correspond to the contralateral tooth.

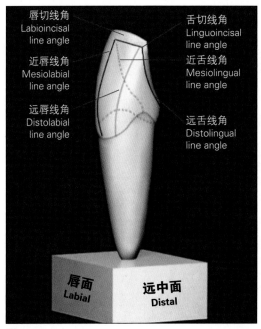

图1–18

12. **点角**：3个相邻牙面相交处形成一点——邻面、唇/颊面和舌面（图1–19）。前牙点角形成了切缘的切角，在制作蜡型或修复体时点角轮廓和位置要恢复到与对侧同名牙一致[6]。

请注意：
- 点角的位置和形态直接影响楔状隙的大小。一般情况下，点角的突度越大，楔状隙也就越大

12. **Point angles** occur at the junction of three surfaces: proximal, facial, and lingual (Fig 1-19). Point angles of anterior teeth form the corners of the incisal edge and should be waxed or restored to correspond in position and contour to the contralateral tooth.[6]

Notice that:
- The point angle location and contour directly affects incisal embrasure size. Typically, the greater the convexity of the point angle, the larger the incisal embrasure will be.

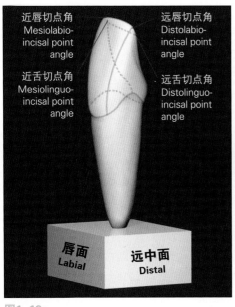

近唇切点角
Mesiolabio-
incisal point
angle

远唇切点角
Distolabio-
incisal point
angle

近舌切点角
Mesiolinguo-
incisal point
angle

远舌切点角
Distolinguo-
incisal point
angle

唇面
Labial

远中面
Distal

图1-19a

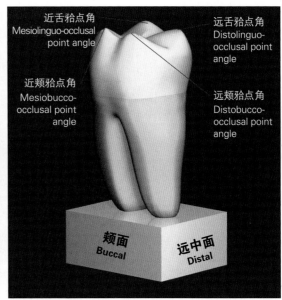

近舌𬌗点角
Mesiolinguo-occlusal
point angle

远舌𬌗点角
Distolinguo-
occlusal point
angle

近颊𬌗点角
Mesiobucco-
occlusal point
angle

远颊𬌗点角
Distobucco-
occlusal point
angle

颊面
Buccal

远中面
Distal

图1-19b

- 颈部邻面形态直接影响颈邻间隙的大小，邻面突度越大，颈邻间隙越小。反之越大
- 邻面接触区位置直接影响颈邻间隙和切楔状隙的大小。颈部接触区越多，切楔状隙越大，颈邻间隙越小

13. **牙面**：前后牙的唇/颊面，其边界为从唇/颊面观来观察到的过渡线角（图1-20）。过渡线角标志着从唇/颊面到近中、颈部、远中和切端的过渡。牙面沿着这些线角的角度向近中面和远中面以及颈部根面倾斜。通常情况下，在唇/颊面切缘部分没有过渡线角。此时，唇/颊面被切缘或𬌗缘包绕[8]。当光线照射到线角时会产生阴影，牙面是唯一反光的区域。因此，牙面的大小决定了人们感知到的唇/颊面大小。过渡线角位置或外形不正确会导致蜡型或修复体即使大小与对侧同名牙一致，也会因为光从一个较小或较大的表面反射而看起来与对侧同名牙大小不一致。

- The proximal surface contour directly affects the cervical embrasure size. The more convex the proximal surface, the smaller the cervical embrasure will be. And the more flat or concave the surface, the larger the embrasure will become.
- Proximal contact location directly affects both cervical and incisal embrasure sizes. The more cervical the proximal contact, the larger the incisal embrasure will be and the smaller the cervical embrasure will be.

13. The **face of a tooth** is the area on the facial surface of anterior and posterior teeth that is bounded by the transitional line angles as viewed from the facial aspect (Fig 1-20). The transitional line angles mark the transition from the facial surface to the mesial, cervical, distal, and incisal surfaces. The tooth surface slopes lingually toward the mesial and distal surfaces and toward the cervical root surface from these line angles. Often, no transitional line angle appears on the incisal portion of the facial surface. In this situation, the face is bounded by the incisal edge or the occlusal tip.[8] Shadows are created as the light strikes the line angles, and the face of the tooth is the only area that reflects light. Therefore, the size of the face of the tooth determines the perceived size of the facial surface. Improper position or contour of transitional line angles will result in a wax-up or a restoration that appears dissimilar, even if it is identical in size to the contralateral tooth, because the light is being reflected from a smaller or larger surface.

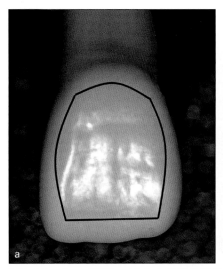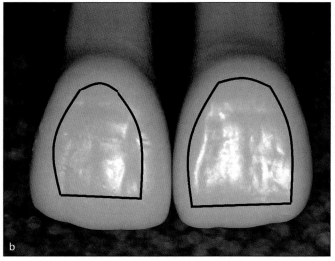

图1-20　（a）牙面。（b）由于线角的位置不同造成光线反射的不同，导致视觉上牙面大小的差异，从而造成外观上的不同

(a) Face of a tooth. *(b)* Differences in the size of the face of the tooth are because of different positions of line angles and result in a dissimilar appearance, given the difference in light reflection.

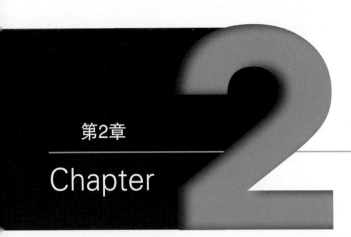

堆塑侧切牙蜡型
Waxing Incisors

上颌侧切牙蜡型堆塑的形态和标准[6-7]

唇面观

从唇面观可以观察到（图2-1a）：

- 外形呈梯形
- 牙冠比中切牙小
- 牙冠比中切牙更圆突
- 远唇线角比近唇线角圆钝，且两个线角的位置和轮廓与对侧同名牙一致
- 远中缘比近中缘更圆突
- 切缘比中切牙更圆钝，其长度、形状、斜度、位置和厚度与对侧同名牙一致
- 切角呈圆弧形（近中侧和远中侧）
- 远中切角比近中切角更圆钝
- 近中接触区位于切1/3与中1/3交界处
- 远中接触区位于中1/3
- 远中切楔状隙比近中切楔状隙大
- 颈邻间隙和切楔状隙与对侧同名牙一致
- 牙冠长度与对侧同名牙一致

Morphology and Criteria for Maxillary Lateral Incisor Wax-Up[6,7]

Labial view

The following can be observed in the labial view (Fig 2-1a):

- Trapezoidal outline.
- Smaller than the central incisor in all dimensions.
- More convex than the central incisor.
- Distolabial line angle more rounded than the mesiolabial line angle, and both line angles consistent in position and contour with the contralateral tooth.
- Distal outline more convex than mesial outline.
- Incisal edge rounded compared with the central incisor and consistent in length, shape, slope, position, and thickness to the contralateral tooth.
- Rounded incisal angles (mesial and distal).
- Disto-incisal angle more rounded than the mesio-incisal angle.
- Mesial contact is at the junction of the incisal and middle thirds.
- Distal contact is at the middle third.
- Disto-incisal embrasure larger than the mesio-incisal embrasure.
- Cervical and incisal embrasures consistent with those of the contralateral tooth.
- Length of the tooth consistent with the contralateral tooth.

舌面观

从舌面观可以观察到（图2-1b）：

- 牙冠向舌侧缩窄
- 舌隆突位于颈1/3。舌隆突的最大突度即舌面外形高点，轮廓和位置与对侧同名牙一致
- 舌窝以切嵴和边缘嵴为界，其深度和宽度与对侧同名牙一致
- 舌窝比上颌中切牙略深
- 边缘嵴比中切牙更明显
- 边缘嵴与邻牙边缘嵴水平相同
- 颈邻间隙和切楔状隙与对侧同名牙一致

Lingual view

The following can be observed in the lingual view (Fig 2-1b):

- Crown tapers lingually.
- Cingulum located in the cervical third. Its maximum convexity represents the lingual height of contour and is consistent in contour and location with the cingulum of the contralateral tooth.
- Lingual fossa is bounded by the well-developed cingulum as well as incisal and marginal ridges and is consistent in depth and width with the contralateral tooth.
- Lingual fossa slightly deeper than that of the maxillary central incisor.
- Marginal ridges more prominent than those of the central incisor.
- Marginal ridges at the same level as the adjacent marginal ridges.
- Cervical and incisal embrasures consistent with those of the contralateral tooth.

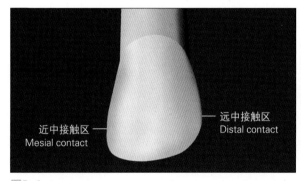

图2-1a

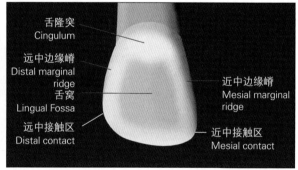

图2-1b

邻面观

从邻面观可以观察到（图2-1c和d）：

- 外形呈三角形
- 唇面和舌面外形高点位于颈1/3，外形高点突出约0.5mm，轮廓与邻牙一致
- 唇舌径与对侧同名牙一致
- 切缘位于牙根唇舌径等分线上

Proximal view

The following can be observed in the proximal views (Figs 2-1c and 2-1d):

- Triangular outline.
- Facial and lingual heights of contours are in the cervical third, and each extends approximately 0.5 mm and is in harmony with the contours of the adjacent teeth.
- Faciolingual dimension of the tooth consistent with that of the contralateral tooth.
- Incisal edge in line with a line bisecting the root labiolingually.

切面观

从切面观可以观察到（图2-1e）：

- 外形呈椭圆形/三角形
- 唇面突度比中切牙更大
- 与中切牙相比，切嵴在唇舌面上更厚，切嵴厚度与对侧同名牙一致
- 舌楔状隙比唇楔状隙宽，二者大小和位置与对侧同名牙一致
- 线角比中切牙更圆钝，与对侧同名牙一致
- 点角的位置和轮廓与对侧同名牙一致

Incisal view

The following can be observed in the incisal view (Fig 2-1e):

- Oval/triangular outline.
- Labial outline more convex than that of central incisor.
- Incisal ridge thicker labiolingually compared with the central incisor and consistent with that of the contralateral tooth.
- Lingual embrasures are wider than the labial embrasures, and both are consistent in size and location with the contralateral tooth.
- Line angles more rounded than those of the central incisor and consistent with the contralateral tooth.
- Point angles consistent in position and contour with the contralateral tooth.

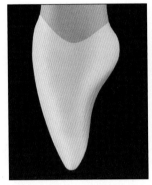 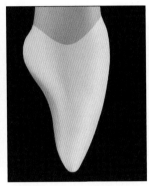 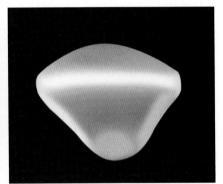

图2-1c 近中邻面观
Mesial view.

图2-1d 远中邻面观
Distal view.

图2-1e

蜡型堆塑入门练习1：#22唇面

通过蜡型堆塑入门练习熟悉蜡型堆塑的技术和方法。练习1是在牙列模型外完成的。

1. 确定牙体预备区的终止线。这条线标志着牙齿预备的终止区域；换句话说，它是缺失牙体组织和剩余牙体组织之间的交界线。唇面蜡型堆塑结束后，终止线应该非常平滑，在图2-2中用红色标出。
2. 使用堆蜡工具，在缺损的唇面堆蜡。从颈部开始（图2-3a），直到蜡层覆盖终止线（图2-3b）。

Introductory Waxing Exercise 1: Facial Surface of #22

Introductory waxing exercises should familiarize you with the wax-addition technique and handling the wax. Exercise 1 is done with the tooth out of the dentoform.

1. Identify the finish line of the prepared area of the tooth. This line marks the termination of the tooth preparation; in other words, it is the junction between the missing tooth structure and the remaining tooth structure. This line should be very smooth when you are finished waxing the facial surface. The finish line is marked in red in Fig 2-2.
2. Using the wax-addition instruments, add wax to the missing facial surface. Start at the cervical area (Fig 2-3a) and continue until the wax covers the finish line (Fig 2-3b).

3. 继续加蜡覆盖整个唇面（图2-4a）。添加更多的蜡以便于雕刻和抛光。在颈1/3处添加更多的蜡，形成唇面和舌面外形高点（图2-4b）。

3. Continue adding wax to cover the entire facial surface (Fig 2-4a). Add excess wax to allow for carving and smoothing. The facial height of contour is created by adding more wax in the cervical third (Fig 2-4b).

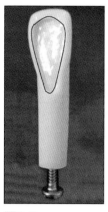 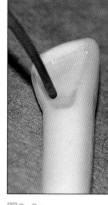 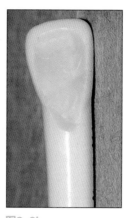 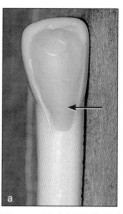 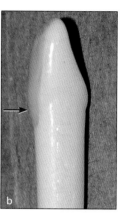

图2-2   图2-3a   图2-3b   图2-4　注意唇面外形高点（箭头所示）
Note facial height of contour (arrows).

4. 清除表面和边缘多余的蜡，将Hollenback雕刻刀部分放在蜡上，部分放在可摘代模上（图2-5）。目的是使蜡与可摘代模的终止线连续，并在可摘代模的界面上形成一个完美的边缘。

5. 当缺损牙体组织延伸至颈缘线的根方时，在唇面复制颈缘线（图2-6）。当缺损牙体组织超过颈缘线，可以使用橡子形抛光器雕刻颈缘线，恢复可摘代模颈缘线的连贯，并且保持颈缘线下方的蜡与周围未预备牙体组织表面光滑连续。蜡型的精修和平整是非常重要的。蜡不能超出缺损牙体组织的边缘（图2-7a）。它应该是非常平滑的且与未预备的牙齿轮廓连续（图2-7b）。平整可以通过雕刻和打磨工具来完成，然后使用一小块尼龙布仔细打磨。

4. Carve away the excess wax on the surface and at the margin by resting the Hollenback carver partly on the wax and partly on the tooth peg (Fig 2-5). The purpose is to make the wax continuous with the finish line of the tooth peg and create a perfect margin at the wax–tooth peg interface.

5. Reproduce the cervical line on the facial surface as the missing tooth structure extends apical to this line (Fig 2-6). This is achieved by carving the cervical line, with the acorn burnisher, continuous with the line on the tooth peg and then carving the wax below the cervical line flat and continuous with the adjacent unprepared tooth surface. Refinement and smoothing of the wax is very important. The wax should not extend beyond the margin of the missing tooth structure (Fig 2-7a). It should be very smooth and continuous with the unprepared tooth contours (Fig 2-7b). Smoothing may be accomplished by carving and burnishing with waxing instruments followed by careful polishing with a small piece of nylon stocking.

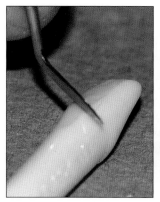 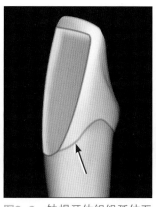 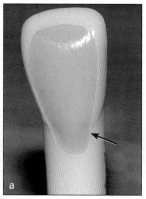

图2-5

图2-6 缺损牙体组织延伸至颈缘线的根方（箭头所示）

Missing tooth structure extends apical to the cervical line *(arrow)*.

图2-7 （a）最终蜡型唇面观。（b）最终蜡型邻面观。注意颈缘线（箭头所示）

Labial *(a)* and proximal *(b)* views of final wax-up. Note the cervical line *(arrow)*.

蜡型堆塑入门练习2：#12近中面

在本练习中，有些堆塑步骤需要将可摘代模放入牙列模型内操作，有些则需要取出可摘代模在牙列模型外操作。使用蜡复制缺失的唇面、舌面、切端和近中面，以及#12的近中接触区和近中边缘嵴（图2-8）。

Introductory Waxing Exercise 2: Proximal Surface of #12

In this exercise, some of the waxing steps are performed with the tooth inside the dentoform and some are performed with the tooth outside of the dentoform. You will reproduce, in wax, part of the labial, lingual, incisal, and mesial surfaces, as well as the mesial contact and marginal ridge of tooth #12 (Fig 2-8).

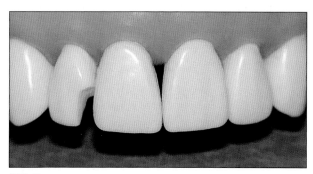

图2-8

1. 确定#12可摘代模终止线（图2-9）。
2. 手握可摘代模，在可摘代模的牙体预备区加蜡，直到覆盖终止线（图2-10）。

1. Identify the finish line on the #12 tooth peg (Fig 2-9).
2. With the tooth peg in your hand, add wax to the prepared area to cover the finish line (Fig 2-10).

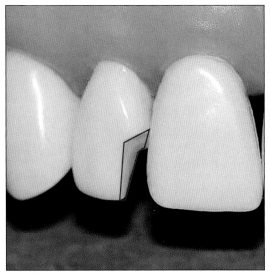
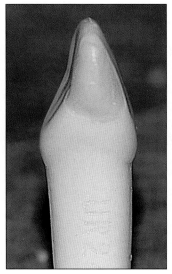
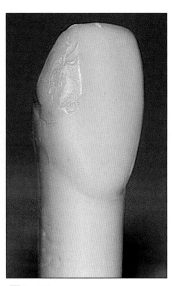

图2-9   图2-10a   图2-10b

3. 将可摘代模放回牙列模型中，并使用铅笔在邻牙（#11）上标记近中接触区位置（图2-11）。接触区通常位于切1/3和中1/3交界处。模仿对侧同名牙接触区位置。

4. 在唇面加蜡，将蜡与#11标记的接触区连接起来（图2-12）。让蜡稍冷却，此时光泽度会消失。

3. Place the tooth peg in the dentoform and mark the proximal contact location on the adjacent tooth (#11) with a pencil (Fig 2-11). The contact is typically at the junction of the incisal and middle thirds. Mimic the contact location on the contralateral side.

4. Apply wax on the labial surface to connect your wax-up with the mark on tooth #11 (Fig 2-12). Allow the wax to cool slightly; the shine should disappear.

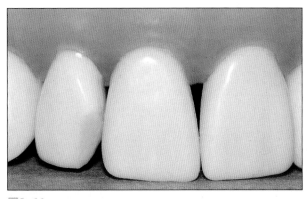
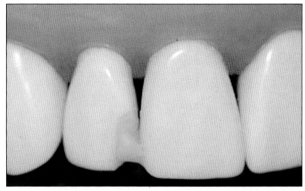

图2-11   图2-12

5. 将可摘代模从牙列模型中取出，填满近中接触区（外形高点）和龈方终止线之间的空隙（图2-13）。

5. Remove the tooth from the dentoform and fill the space between the proximal contact (height of contour) and the gingival finish line (Fig 2-13).

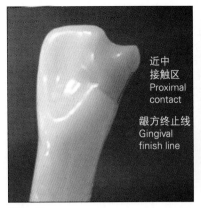
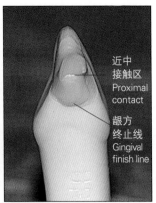

图2-13a

图2-13b

6. 切除近中接触区多余的蜡，形成平坦的近中邻面。切除超出终止线的多余的蜡（图2-14）。

6. Carve the wax cervical to the contact to create a flat proximal surface. Carve away any excess beyond the finish line (Fig 2-14).

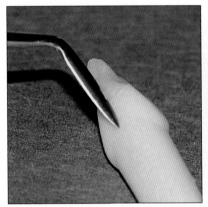
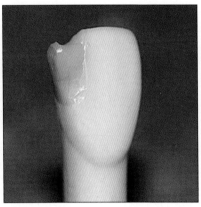
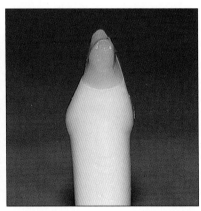

图2-14a

图2-14b

图2-14c

7. 将可摘代模放回牙列模型中，并确认近中接触区的密合情况和位置（图2-15）。如果在雕刻过程中失去接触，需额外加蜡。

8. 在唇面加蜡，完成唇面轮廓（图2-16）。

9. 在舌面加蜡，完成舌面轮廓（图2-17）。

7. Return the tooth to the dentoform and confirm the closure and position of the proximal contact (Fig 2-15). Additional wax should be added if the contact was lost during carving.

8. Apply wax to complete the facial surface (Fig 2-16).

9. Apply wax to complete the lingual surface (Fig 2-17).

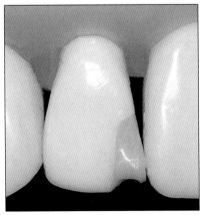
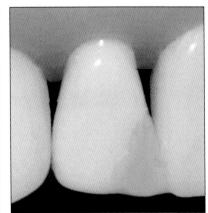
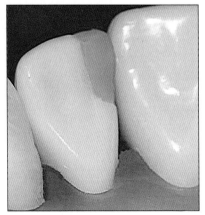

图2-15

图2-16

图2-17

10. 保持可摘代模在牙列模型中，使用Hollenback雕刻刀平齐蜡型切缘（图2-18）。

11. 通过轻轻地在#12和#11之间的邻面接触区加蜡，形成近中切楔状隙（图2-19）。注意#12近中切角略圆，与远中切角相比突度较小。因此，近中切楔状隙比远中切楔状隙小。

12. 使用Hollenback雕刻刀切除唇面和唇面终止线处多余的蜡（图2-20）。

10. With the tooth in the dentoform, level the incisal edge of the wax up with the incisal edge of the tooth peg using the Hollenback carver (Fig 2-18).

11. Create the mesio-incisal embrasure by gently carving the wax incisal to the proximal contact between #12 and #11 (Fig 2-19). Notice that the mesio-incisal angle of #12 is only slightly rounded and is less convex compared with the disto-incisal angle. Therefore, the mesio-incisal embrasure is smaller than the disto-incisal embrasure.

12. Carve excess wax at the labial surface and the labial finish line with the Hollenback carver (Fig 2-20).

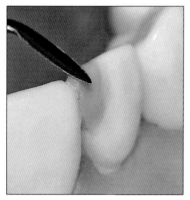

图2-18

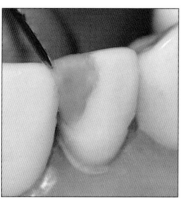

图2-19

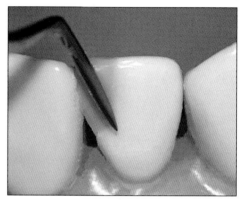

图2-20

13. 使用超细黑色记号笔在蜡型上标出近唇线角作为可摘代模预备的位置，标记线角有助于预先定位其位置。沿着标记的线向舌面进行雕刻，形成线角（图2-21）。当完成雕刻后，轻轻刮除黑色标记线。

13. Mark the location of the mesiolabial line angle on the wax-up with an ultrafine-point black marker as a continuation to the one on the unprepared surface of the tooth peg. Marking the line angle helps to preserve its position. Carve away from the line you marked toward the lingual surface to create the line angle (Fig 2-21). The black mark can be carved gently when you are done.

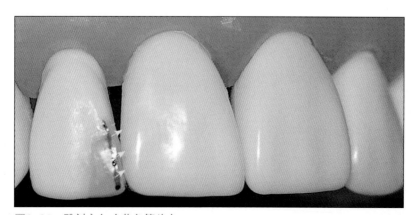

图2-21 雕刻方向（黄色箭头）
The direction of carving (yellow arrows).

14. 切除舌面多余的蜡（图2-22）。这一步的关键是使可摘代模上堆塑的蜡型表面平整。避免在下一步雕刻舌面解剖结构和边缘嵴时去除过多的蜡。

15. 使用盘-爪状雕刻刀雕刻出舌窝（图2-23）。一旦舌窝形成，相邻边缘嵴和切嵴通过最小限度地修形和抛光来强调。

14. Carve the excess wax at the lingual surface (Fig 2-22). The goal at this point is to level the wax surface with that of the tooth peg. Avoid removing too much wax to allow carving the lingual anatomy and the marginal ridge in the next step.

15. Use the small discoid-cleoid carver to carve the lingual fossa (Fig 2-23). Once the fossa is created, the adjacent marginal and incisal ridges are easily emphasized with minimal contouring and polishing.

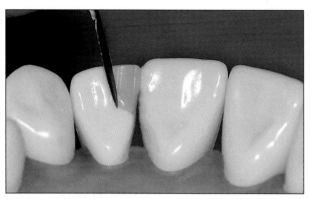
图2-22

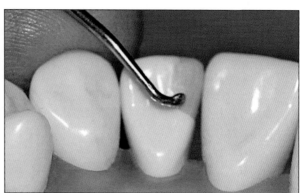
图2-23

16. 分别从唇面观和舌面观检查最终的堆蜡效果。近唇线角、近唇切点角和近中切楔状隙均应与对侧同名牙一致（图2-24）。唇面和舌面形态应与对侧同名牙一致，并与邻牙协调。

16. Check the final wax-up from the labial and lingual views. The mesiolabial line angle, mesiolabio-incisal point angle, and mesio-incisal embrasure should all conform with those of the contralateral tooth (Fig 2-24). The facial and lingual contours should conform to the contralateral tooth and be harmonious with the adjacent teeth.

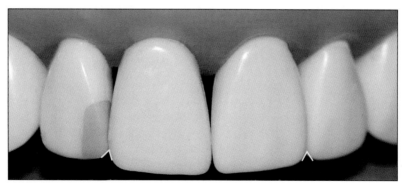
图2-24

17. 使用尼龙布抛光蜡型。检查边缘是否与可摘代模连续，蜡型是否光滑，牙列模型上是否有多余的蜡屑（图2-25）。

17. Smooth and polish your wax-up with a nylon stocking. Check that the margins are continuous with the tooth peg, the wax-up is nicely polished, and there are no wax flakes on the dentoform (Fig 2-25).

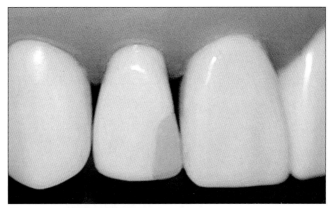

图2-25a　最终蜡型唇面观
Labial view of the final wax-up.

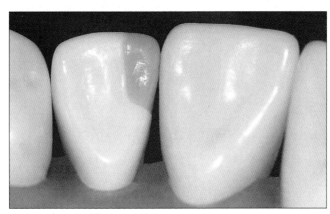

图2-25b　最终蜡型舌面观
Lingual view of the final wax-up.

下颌侧切牙全冠蜡型堆塑的形态和标准[6-7]

唇面观

从唇面观可以观察到（图2-26a）：

- 外形呈梯形
- 下颌侧切牙的近远中径比下颌中切牙大
- 牙冠不如下颌中切牙那样近中缘与远中缘对称
- 远唇线角比近唇线角略圆钝，两个线角在位置和轮廓上都与对侧同名牙一致
- 切缘笔直，其长度、形状、斜度、位置和厚度与对侧同名牙一致
- 远中缘比近中缘更圆突
- 近中切角接近90°；远中切角略圆钝

Morphology and Criteria for Mandibular Lateral Incisor Full-Crown Wax-Up[6,7]

Labial view

The following can be observed in the labial view (Fig 2-26a):

- Trapezoidal outline.
- Mesiodistal dimension greater than that of the mandibular central incisor.
- Crown not bilaterally symmetric like the mandibular central incisor.
- Distolabial line angle slightly more rounded than the mesiolabial line angle, and both line angles consistent in position and contour with the contralateral tooth.
- Incisal edge is straight and consistent in length, shape, slope, position, and thickness to the contralateral tooth.
- Distal outline more convex than mesial outline.
- Mesio-incisal angle approaches 90 degrees; disto-incisal angle slightly more rounded.

- 近中和远中接触区位于牙冠的切1/3处
- 远中接触区距切角略远，但仍位于切1/3内
- 远中切楔状隙比近中切楔状隙略大
- 切楔状隙和颈邻间隙的大小、位置与对侧同名牙一致
- 切颈径（即牙冠长度）与对侧同名牙一致

- Mesial and distal contacts located at the incisal third of the crown.
- Distal contact area slightly more cervical but still in the incisal third.
- Disto-incisal embrasure is slightly larger than the mesio-incisal embrasure.
- Incisal and cervical embrasures are consistent in size and location with those of the contralateral tooth.
- The incisocervical dimension (ie, length of the tooth) is consistent with the contralateral tooth.

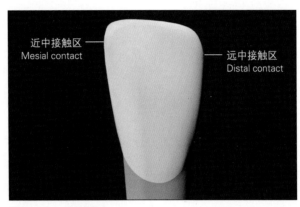

近中接触区
Mesial contact

远中接触区
Distal contact

图2-26a　唇面观
Labial view.

舌面观

从舌面观可以观察到（图2-26b）：

- 牙冠向舌侧缩窄
- 舌隆突位于颈1/3。舌隆突的最大突度即舌面外形高点，其轮廓和位置与对侧同名牙一致
- 虽然下颌侧切牙的舌窝比中切牙略明显，但所有下颌切牙的舌窝仍窄浅，其深度和宽度与对侧同名牙一致
- 近中和远中边缘嵴比下颌中切牙更明显，与邻牙边缘嵴处于同一水平
- 切楔状隙和颈邻间隙的大小、位置与对侧同名牙一致

邻面观

从邻面观可以观察到（图2-26c和d）：

- 外形呈三角形
- 唇面略突，舌面略突的切嵴和舌隆突之间的凹陷处为舌窝

Lingual view

The following can be observed in the lingual view (Fig 2-26b):

- Crown tapers lingually.
- Cingulum located in the cervical third. Its maximum convexity represents the lingual height of contour and is consistent in contour and location with the cingulum of the contralateral tooth.
- Lingual fossa of the mandibular lateral incisor slightly more evident than in the central incisor, but it is still shallow as all mandibular incisor fossae and is consistent in depth and width to the contralateral tooth.
- Mesial and distal marginal ridges more pronounced than those of the mandibular central incisor and at the same level as the adjacent marginal ridges.
- Incisal and cervical embrasures consistent in size and location with those of the contralateral tooth.

Proximal view

The following can be observed in the proximal views (Fig 2-26c and 2-26d):

- Triangular outline.
- Labial surface convex; lingual surface convex incisally and cervically but concave between the two areas where the lingual fossa is.

- 唇舌径比下颌中切牙大，与对侧同名牙一致
- 唇面和舌面外形高点位于颈1/3，外形高点突出约0.5mm，轮廓与邻牙一致
- 近中邻面比远中邻面略长
- 切嵴略偏于牙根唇舌径等分线的舌侧

- Labiolingual dimension greater than that of the mandibular central incisor and consistent with that of the contralateral tooth.
- Facial and lingual heights of contour located at the cervical third of the tooth, and each extends 0.5 mm and is in harmony with the contours of the adjacent teeth.
- Mesial surface tends to be slightly longer than the distal surface.
- Incisal ridge slightly lingual to a line bisecting the root labiolingually.

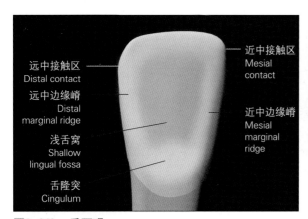

图2-26b　舌面观
Lingual view.

远中接触区 Distal contact
远中边缘嵴 Distal marginal ridge
浅舌窝 Shallow lingual fossa
舌隆突 Cingulum
近中接触区 Mesial contact
近中边缘嵴 Mesial marginal ridge

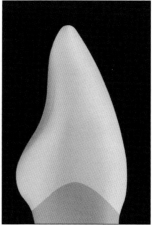

图2-26c　近中邻面观
Mesial view.

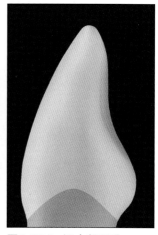

图2-26d　远中邻面观
Distal view.

切面观

从切面观可以观察到（图2-26e）：

- 外形呈椭圆形/三角形
- 唇舌径比近远中径大
- 牙冠两侧不对称
- 切嵴在牙根上向远舌侧旋转，与对侧同名牙一致
- 近远中唇面突度比中切牙更大
- 近唇线角和远唇线角比中切牙更圆突，并与对侧同名牙一致
- 所有点角的位置和轮廓与对侧同名牙一致
- 舌窝比唇窝宽，二者大小和位置与对侧同名牙一致

Incisal view

The following can be observed in the incisal view (Fig 2-26e):

- Oval/triangular outline.
- Labiolingual dimension greater than the mesiodistal dimension.
- Crown not bilaterally symmetric.
- Incisal ridge rotated distolingually on the root and consistent with that of the contralateral tooth.
- Labial surface more convex mesiodistally than that of the central incisor.
- Mesiolabial and distolabial line angles more convex than those of the central incisors and consistent with those of the contralateral tooth.
- All point angles consistent in position and contour with those of the contralateral tooth.
- Lingual embrasures wider than the labial embrasures, and both are consistent in size and location with those of the contralateral tooth.

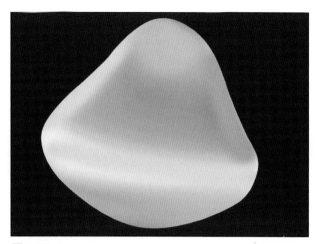

图2-26e

#32全冠蜡型堆塑步骤

全冠蜡型堆塑需要注意更多的技巧和细节，因为可摘代模上没有正常的牙体组织来引导。可以参照邻牙和对侧同名牙。观察对侧同名牙#42解剖形态（图2-27）。以其为目标制作#42的镜像。从牙列模型中取出#32可摘代模。有些堆塑步骤需要将可摘代模放入牙列模型内操作，有些则需要取出可摘代模在牙列模型外操作。在本练习中，只需使用下颌牙列模型。按照以下步骤进行全冠蜡型堆塑。

Waxing Steps for Tooth #32 Full-Crown Wax-Up

Waxing full-crowns requires more skill and attention to detail because you do not have the remaining tooth structure on the tooth peg to guide you. Your main guides are the adjacent teeth and the contralateral tooth. Notice the anatomy of the contralateral tooth #42 (Fig 2-27). Your goal is to create a mirror image of tooth #42. Unscrew #32 from your dentoform so you can place the tooth peg. Some of the waxing steps are performed inside the dentoform and some are performed outside the dentoform. Only the mandibular dentoform arch is used in this exercise. Follow these steps to wax your first full-crown.

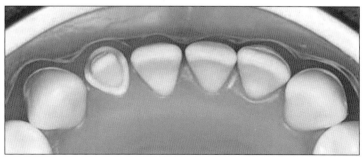

图2-27

1. 形成初始蜡层。

- 手握可摘代模，开始在可摘代模的牙体预备区加蜡（图2-28a）。蜡层厚度均匀，覆盖整个预备区（图2-28b），不留空隙

- 延长蜡层超过终止线（图2-28c），以确保蜡层边缘没有缺陷。在下一步清除终止线外多余的蜡

- 使用Hollenback雕刻刀雕刻蜡型，使之与终止线平齐且轮廓合适，以实现与可摘代模的平滑过渡（图2-28d和e）

1. Establish the initial layer of wax.

- With the tooth peg in your hand, start adding wax to cover the prepared area of the tooth peg (Fig 2-28a). The wax should be of even thickness and cover the entire prepared area (Fig 2-28b). There should be no voids in the wax.

- Extend the wax past the finish line (Fig 2-28c). This is done to ensure that the wax is not deficient at the margin. Excess wax at the finish line is removed in the next part of this step.

- Use the Hollenback carver to carve the wax flush with the finish line and with the proper contour to achieve a smooth transition with the tooth peg (Figs 2-28d and 2-28e).

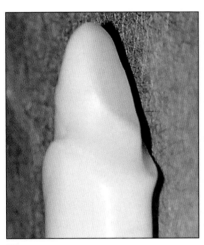

图2-28a

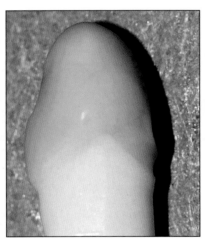

图2-28b

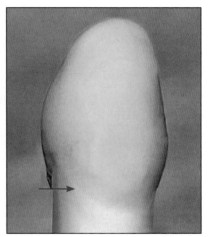

图2-28c

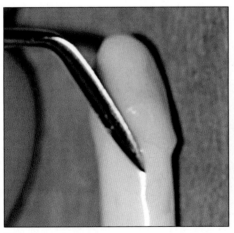

图2-28d

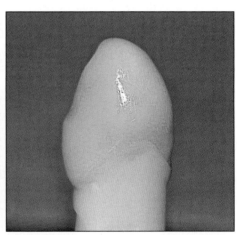

图2-28e

2. 形成邻接关系。

• 将可摘代模放回牙列模型中，并使用铅笔在邻牙上标记颊面接触区的位置（图2-29a）。邻面接触区位于#32的切1/3，注意要在邻牙上做标记（近中接触区标记在#33，远中接触区标记在#31，两个接触区都位于牙冠切1/3处）。还可以将未预备的#32放回牙列模型中并标记位置或模仿对侧同名牙的接触区位置

• 添加蜡锥，将蜡型和邻牙上的标记连接起来。继续加蜡，直到蜡锥与标记牢固接触（图2-29b和c）。在蜡完全冷却之前，不要将蜡型从牙列模型中取出。蜡锥应与邻牙外形高点（即最大突度）连接。接触区部位多余的蜡可以在步骤3中雕刻清除

2. Establish the proximal contacts.

• Return the tooth to the dentoform and mark the typical location for the proximal contacts on the buccal surface of the adjacent teeth with a pencil (Fig 2-29a). Proximal contacts of tooth #32 are located in the incisal third. Remember that you are marking the location on the adjacent teeth (ie, mesial contact of #33 and distal contact of #31, which in this case are also located in the incisal third). You can either replace the unprepared tooth #32 in the dentoform to mark the location or mimic the proximal contact location on the contralateral side.

• Add wax cones to connect your wax-up with the marks on the adjacent teeth. Continue adding wax until the cones make firm contact with the marks (Figs 2-29b and 2-29c). Do not remove the tooth from the dentoform until the wax cools completely. The wax cones should contact the adjacent teeth at their height of contour (ie, maximum convexity). Excess wax away from the location of the contact can be carved in step 3.

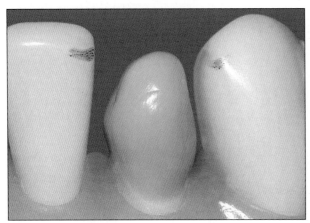

图2-29a

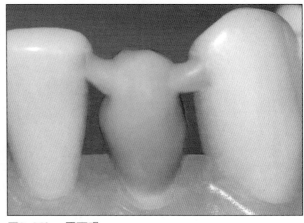

图2-29b　唇面观
Labial view.

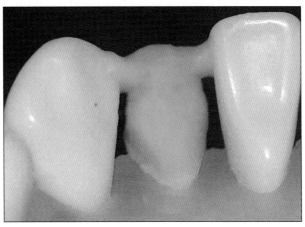

图2-29c　舌面观
Lingual view.

3. 形成邻面接触区。

- 将可摘代模从牙列模型中取出，继续在邻面接触区加蜡至龈方终止线，保持蜡表面相对平坦（图2-30a和b）

- 使用Hollenback雕刻刀雕刻邻面，由颈缘至邻面接触区修平表面（图2-30c）。应注意避免雕刻接触区。邻面应在切龈向和唇舌向的龈方至接触区保持相对平坦

3. Wax the proximal surface.

- Remove the tooth from the dentoform, and add wax to connect the proximal contact to the gingival finish line, keeping the wax relatively flat (Figs 2-30a and 2-30b).

- Use your Hollenback carver to carve the proximal surfaces flat cervical to the contact (Fig 2-30c). Care should be taken to avoid carving the contact. Proximal surfaces are relatively flat labiolingually and incisocervically between the contact area and the cervical line.

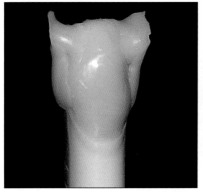 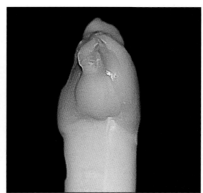 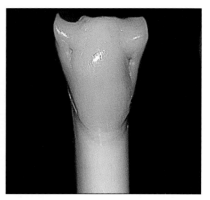

图2-30a 图2-30b 图2-30c

4. 形成切缘。

- 将可摘代模放回牙列模型中，在切缘部分加蜡，形成切缘（图2-31a）。每次加蜡时都要拖动，从邻牙开始。理想情况下，下颌侧切牙比下颌中切牙略长。然而，在该牙列模型上，对侧的下颌侧切牙略短。尽量模仿对侧同名牙的长度，即使它偏离了理想长度——就像在口腔中修复牙齿那样

- 使用Hollenback雕刻刀调整切缘的长度（图2-31b）。楔状隙可在这一步雕刻或在完成唇面、舌面堆塑后雕刻

- 保持可摘代模在牙列模型中，使用Hollenback雕刻刀雕刻切楔状隙（图2-31c~e）。模仿对侧同名牙的楔状隙。远中切角比近中切角更圆钝，因此远切楔状隙比近中切楔状隙略大。在堆蜡完成后，可以通过加蜡或雕刻点角进一步调整楔状隙

4. Establish the incisal edge.

- Return the tooth to the dentoform and add wax to the incisal part of your wax-up to form the incisal edge (Fig 2-31a). The wax is dragged while being added between the proximal ends of the incisal part of the wax-up. Ideally, the mandibular lateral incisor is slightly longer than the mandibular central incisor. However, on the dentoform shown here, the mandibular lateral incisor on the contralateral side is slightly shorter. You should always mimic the length of the contralateral tooth—even if it deviates from the ideal—just as you would when restoring teeth in the mouth.

- Adjust the length of the incisal edge with the Hollenback carver (Fig 2-31b). Embrasures can be carved following incisal edge adjustment or after the labial or lingual surfaces are waxed.

- With the tooth in the dentoform, carve the incisal embrasures with the Hollenback carver (Figs 2-31c to 2-31e). Mimic the embrasures on the contralateral side. Remember that the disto-incisal angle is more round than the mesio-incisal angle, and the disto-incisal embrasure is slightly larger than the mesio-incisal embrasure. Further adjustment of the embrasures is done after finishing the wax-up by wax addition or carving at the point angles.

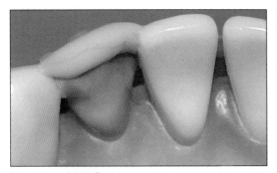
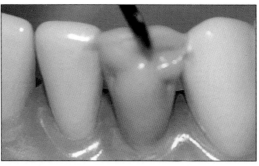

图2-31a 切面观
Incisal view.

图2-31b

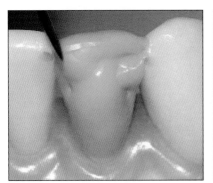
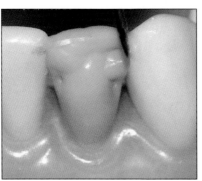
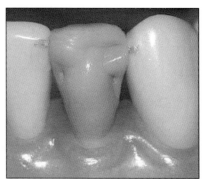

图2-31c

图2-31d

图2-31e

5. 堆塑唇面。

- 保持可摘代模在牙列模型中，在唇面加蜡，完成唇面轮廓（图2-32a）。在颈1/3处添加更多的蜡，形成外形高点。然后通过连接近中边界、远中边界和外形高点形成相应的线角

- 唇面塑形。使用超细黑色记号笔粗略标出唇面外形高点和过渡线角的位置（图2-32b；过渡线角之间的部分称为牙面）。可以使用铅笔在对侧同名牙上画出牙面形态，以帮助我们复制出线角和唇面外形高点，从而得到蜡型牙面的精确尺寸

- 将可摘代模从牙列模型中取出，在标记区之内雕刻，保持标记位置的线角和外形高点（图2-32c）。轻柔雕刻，以避免产生无法抛光的凹痕

5. Wax the labial surface.

- With the tooth in the dentoform, add a layer of wax to the labial surface to complete the labial contour (Fig 2-32a). Apply more wax at the cervical third where the height of contour is located. Apply more wax at the mesial and distal boundaries where the line angles are located.

- Labial surface carving. With the ultrafine-point black marker, roughly mark the location of the labial height of contour and the transitional line angles (Fig 2-32b; The part of the tooth between the transitional line angles is called the *face of the tooth*). You may mark the face of the tooth on the contralateral tooth with a pencil to help you duplicate the exact location of the line angles and labial height of contour and therefore the exact size of the face of the tooth.

- Remove the tooth from the dentoform and carve between the marks and outside the marks, keeping the line angles and the height of contour at the marked location (Fig 2-32c). Carving is done very gently to avoid creating gouges that cannot be polished.

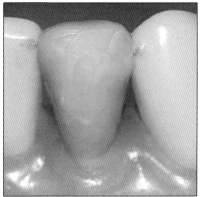

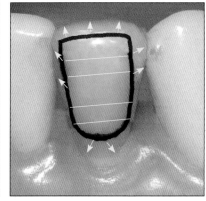

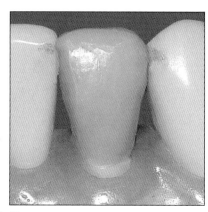

图2-32a

图2-32b 雕刻方向（黄色箭头和线条） 图2-32c

The direction of carving(yellow arrows and lines).

6. 堆塑舌面

• 保持可摘代模在牙列模型中，舌面加一层蜡，完成舌面轮廓。在颈1/3处添加更多的蜡，形成舌隆突。在近中边界和远中边界添加更多的蜡，形成近中边缘嵴和远中边缘嵴（图2-33a）

• 堆塑舌面。使用超细黑色记号笔标记舌窝边界（模仿对侧同名牙舌窝形态）（图2-33b）。将可摘代模从牙列模型中取出，使用盘-爪状雕刻刀的小工作尖雕刻舌窝（图2-33c）。在雕刻舌窝后，所有周边的凸起（边缘嵴、舌隆突、切嵴）可以通过最小限度地修形和抛光来强调

6. Wax the lingual surface.

• With the tooth in the dentoform, add a layer of wax to the lingual surface to complete the lingual contour. Apply more wax at the cervical third to form the cingulum. Apply more wax at the mesial and distal boundaries to form the marginal ridges (Fig 2-33a).

• Lingual surface carving. Mark the lingual fossa boundaries with the ultrafine-point black marker (mimic the lingual fossa of the contralateral tooth) (Fig 2-33b). Remove the tooth from the dentoform and carve the lingual fossa with the small discoid-cleoid carver (Fig 2-33c). All the surrounding elevations (marginal ridges, cingulum, and incisal ridge) can be emphasized easily with minimal contouring and polishing after carving the lingual fossa.

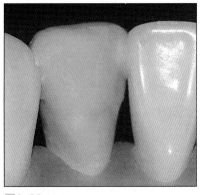

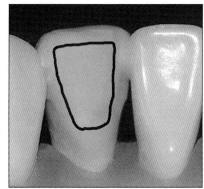

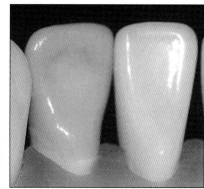

图2-33a

图2-33b

图2-33c

7. 完成最终的雕刻和修形。

• 从不同角度检查线角、点角、楔状隙、切缘、邻面接触区、舌面解剖结构、外形高点和终止线。根据需要进行加蜡和雕刻，来最终实现蜡型形态与对侧同名牙一致、与邻牙和谐（图2-34）

7. Complete the final carving and contouring.

• Line angles, point angles, embrasures, incisal edge, proximal contacts, lingual anatomy, heights of contour, and finish line are all checked from different views, and wax addition and carving are done as needed to achieve a final wax-up that is consistent with the contralateral tooth and harmonious with the adjacent teeth (Fig 2-34).

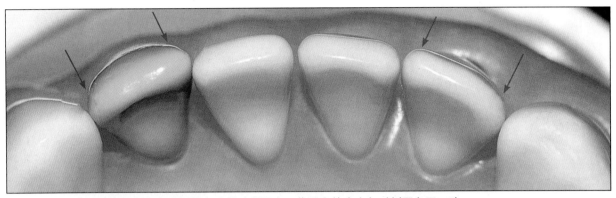

图2-34a　最好从切面观来观察唇侧线角（箭头所示），位置和轮廓应与对侧同名牙一致
Labial line angles *(arrows)* are best visualized from the incisal view and should conform in position and contour with those of the contralateral tooth.

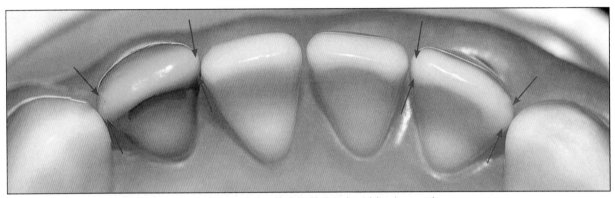

图2-34b　最好从切面观来观察点角（箭头所示），位置和轮廓应与对侧同名牙一致
Point angles *(arrows)* are best visualized from the incisal view and should conform in position and contour to those of the contralateral tooth.

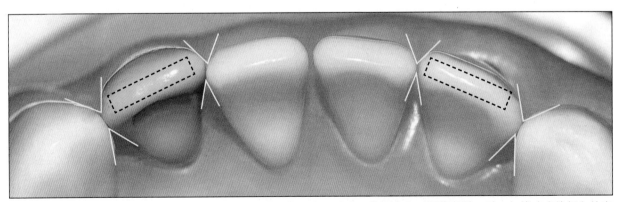

图2-34c　从切面观来观察唇楔状隙和舌楔状隙（黄色标记），大小、位置应与对侧楔状隙一致。切缘（虚线框）的宽度和厚度应与对侧同名牙一致
The labial and lingual embrasures *(in yellow)* are visualized from the incisal view and should match the contralateral embrasures in size and location. The width and thickness of the incisal edge *(dotted boxes)* should conform to that of the contralateral tooth.

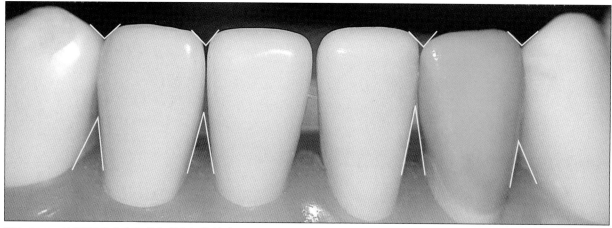

图2-34d 从唇面观或舌面观来观察切楔状隙和颈邻间隙（黄色标记）。远中切楔状隙比近中切楔状隙略大，远中切角更圆钝

Incisal and cervical embrasures *(in yellow)* are visualized from the labial or lingual view. The disto-incisal embrasure is slightly larger than the mesio-incisal embrasure, given the more rounded disto-incisal point angle.

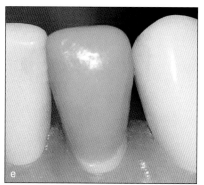
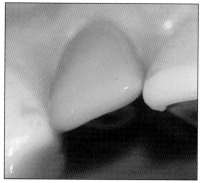
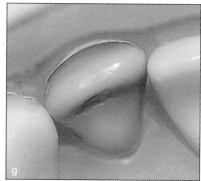

图2-34e~g 在适当光源下，从各个面仔细检查接触区的密合情况和位置（切龈向和唇舌向）。即使在口内对侧同名牙邻面未与邻牙接触，蜡型的接触区都要恢复正常接触区

The proximal contact closure and position (incisogingival and labiolingual) is checked by carefully inspecting the wax-up from all views with proper illumination. Notice that even if your contralateral tooth has an open contact, your wax-up must have a closed contact.

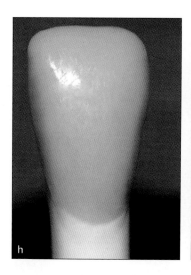
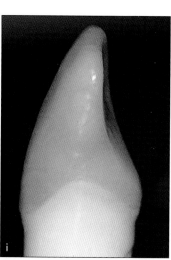

图2-34h和i

将蜡型从牙列模型中取出，确认邻牙与蜡型之间的邻接面是平滑过渡的。和未预备的#32比对外形轮廓的大小

Remove the wax-up from the dento- form, and verify that the transition from the unprepared tooth to the wax is smooth and there is no defi-ciency at the margin. You can hold the unprepared #32 tooth adjacent to your wax-up and compare contours.

8. 完成最终的平整和抛光。

- 使用雕刻刀修平表面，再使用尼龙布轻轻
抛光。这应该会让蜡型看起来更漂亮（图
2-35）。应避免长时间地打磨，因为这会改
变牙体的结构。为了避免破坏蜡型，抛光时勿
过度加压。使用注射器吹气或刷子清除蜡型和
牙列模型上多余的蜡屑

8. Complete final smoothing and polishing.
- Plane the surface with a carver and buff lightly with a nylon stocking. This should give your wax-up a nice polished appearance (Fig 2-35). Avoid lengthy polishing as it may change the tooth anatomy. Use only gentle pressure to avoid breaking your wax-up. Remove wax flakes from your wax-up and the dentoform using the airway syringe or a brush.

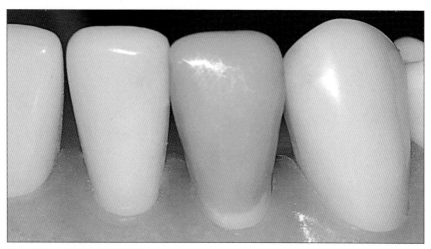

图2-35a 最终蜡型唇面观
Labial view of the final wax-up.

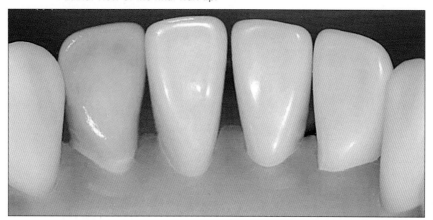

图2-35b 最终蜡型舌面观
Lingual view of the final wax-up.

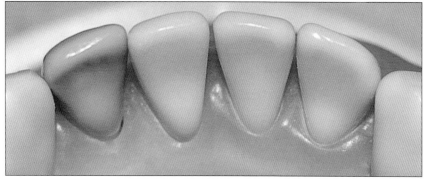

图2-35c 最终蜡型切面观
Incisal view of the final wax-up.

上颌中切牙全冠蜡型堆塑的形态和标准[6-7]

唇面观

从唇面观可以观察到（图2-36a）：

- 外形呈梯形
- 在所有前牙中近远中径最宽
- 切颈径比近远中径大，与相邻中切牙一致
- 上颌中切牙唇面近远中、颈部光滑凸起
- 两叶之间存在两个宽的唇发育沟，分别称为近唇发育沟、远唇发育沟
- 近唇线角略凸
- 远唇线角比近唇线角更圆突
- 近中切角几乎成90°
- 远中切角比近中切角更圆钝
- 近中接触区位于近中切角靠近切1/3处
- 远中接触区位于切1/3和中1/3交界处

舌面观

从舌面观可以观察到（图2-36b）：

- 舌面比唇面窄，近远中边缘嵴向舌面逐渐变细（即舌向聚合）
- 舌窝以近远中边缘嵴、舌隆突和切嵴为界。舌窝近远中向、切颈向呈凹陷状，在宽度和深度上与相邻中切牙一致
- 切嵴突出，与近远中边缘嵴相连
- 舌隆突凸起，在高度和位置上与相邻中切牙一致
- 与邻牙边缘嵴处于同一水平
- 切楔状隙和颈邻间隙与相邻中切牙一致

Morphology and Criteria for Maxillary Central Incisor Full-Crown Wax-Up[6,7]

Labial view

The following can be observed in the labial view (Fig 2-36a):

- Trapezoidal outline.
- Widest anterior tooth mesiodistally.
- Cervico-incisal dimension greater than mesiodistal dimension and consistent with the adjacent central incisor.
- Labial surface of maxillary central incisor smooth and convex mesiodistally and cervico-incisally.
- Two wide labial developmental depressions exist between the lobes and are called the *mesiolabial* and *distolabial developmental depressions*.
- Mesiolabial line angle slightly convex.
- Distolabial line angle more convex than the mesiolabial line angle.
- Mesio-incisal angle almost 90 degrees.
- Disto-incisal angle more rounded than the mesio-incisal angle.
- Mesial contact area at the incisal third of the crown, near the mesioincisal angle.
- Distal contact area at the junction of incisal and middle thirds of the crown.

Lingual view

The following can be observed in the lingual view (Fig 2-36b):

- Lingual surface narrower than the labial surface given that the mesial and distal walls taper toward the lingual aspect (ie, *lingual convergence*).
- Lingual fossa bounded by the prominent marginal ridges, the cingulum, and the incisal ridge. It is concave mesiodistally and incisocervically and consistent with the fossa of the adjacent central incisor in width and depth.
- Incisal ridge raised and continuous with mesial and distal marginal ridges.
- Cingulum prominent and convex and consistent with the cingulum of the adjacent central incisor in contour and location.
- Marginal ridges at the same level as the adjacent marginal ridges.
- Incisal and cervical embrasures consistent with those of the adjacent central incisor.

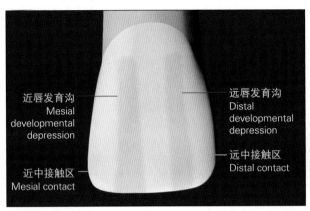

图2-36a

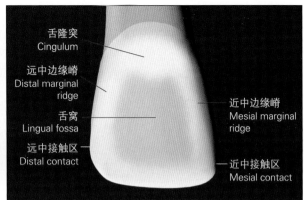

图2-36b

邻面观

从邻面观可以观察到（图2-36c和d）：

- 外形呈三角形
- 唇面轮廓外凸
- 舌面轮廓自舌隆突处凸起到舌窝处凹陷
- 切缘位于牙根唇舌径等分线上
- 唇面和舌面外形高点位于颈1/3，外形高点突出约0.5mm，轮廓与相邻中切牙一致
- 唇舌径与相邻中切牙一致

切面观

从切面观可以观察到（图2-36e）：

- 外形呈三角形
- 近远中径比唇舌径略大
- 舌隆突略偏远中，位置和轮廓与相邻中切牙一致
- 近远中唇面略凸
- 可见两个唇发育沟，且均与相邻中切牙一致
- 近唇线角和远唇线角比舌侧线角更明显。所有线角在位置和轮廓上都与相邻中切牙一致
- 所有点角在位置和轮廓上与相邻中切牙一致
- 舌楔状隙比唇楔状隙宽，大小、位置与相邻中切牙一致

Proximal view

The following can be observed in the proximal views (Figs 2-36c and 2-36d):

- Triangular outline.
- Labial outline convex.
- Lingual outline starts convex at the cingulum then becomes concave at the lingual fossa.
- Incisal edge in line with the line bisecting the root labiolingually.
- Labial and lingual heights of contour are at the cervical third, extend 0.5 mm, and are consistent with those of the adjacent central incisor.
- Faciolingual dimension of the tooth consistent with that of the adjacent central incisor.

Incisal view

The following can be observed in the incisal view (Fig 2-36e):

- Triangular outline.
- Mesiodistal dimension slightly greater than labiolingual dimension.
- Cingulum slightly off center to the distal and is consistent in location and contour to that of the adjacent central incisor.
- Labial surface slightly convex mesiodistally.
- Two labial developmental depressions visible, and both are consistent with the adjacent central incisor.
- Mesiolabial and distolabial line angles more prominent than the lingual line angles. All line angles consistent in position and contour with those of the adjacent central incisor.
- All point angles consistent in position and contour with those of the adjacent central incisor.
- Lingual embrasures wider than the labial embrasures, and both consistent in size and location with the adjacent central incisor.

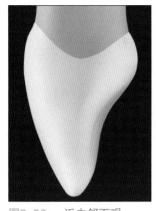 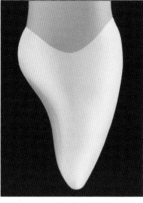 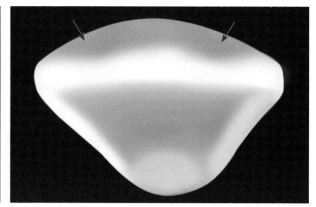

图2-36c 近中邻面观
Mesial view.

图2-36d 远中邻面观
Distal view.

图2-36e 近唇发育沟、远唇发育沟（箭头所示）
Mesial and distal developmental depressions *(arrows)*.

#21全冠蜡型堆塑步骤

从牙列模型中取出#21可摘代模（图2-37）。有些堆塑步骤需要将可摘代模放入牙列模型内操作，有些则需要取出可摘代模在牙列模型外操作。在本练习中只需使用上颌牙列模型。

Waxing Steps for Tooth #21 Full-Crown Wax-Up

Unscrew #21 from your dentoform so you can place the tooth peg (Fig 2-37). Some of the waxing steps are performed inside the dentoform and some are performed outside. Only the maxillary dentoform arch is used in this exercise.

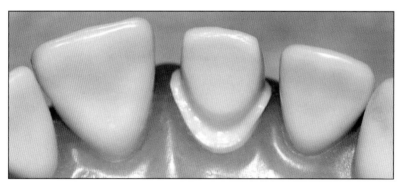

图2-37

1. 形成初始蜡层。
- 手握可摘代模，开始在可摘代模的牙体预备区加蜡（图2-38a和b）。蜡层厚度均匀，覆盖整个预备区，不留空隙
- 延长蜡层超过终止线，以确保蜡层边缘没有缺陷（图2-38c）
- 使用Hollenback雕刻刀雕刻蜡型，使之与终止线平齐且轮廓合适，以实现与可摘代模的平滑过渡（图2-38d）

1. Establish an initial layer of wax.
- With the tooth peg in your hand, start adding wax to cover the prepared area of the tooth peg (Figs 2-38a and 2-38b). The wax should be of even thickness and cover the entire prepared area. There should be no voids in the wax.
- Extend the wax past the finish line to ensure that the wax is not deficient at the margin (Fig 2-38c).
- Use the Hollenback carver to carve the wax flush with the finish line and with the proper contour to achieve a smooth transition with the tooth peg (Fig 2-38d).

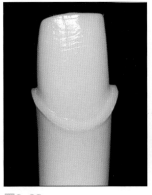
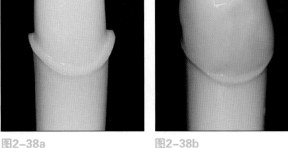
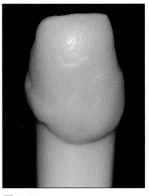
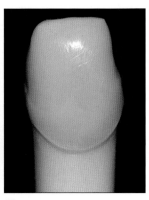

图2-38a　　　　　　图2-38b　　　　　　图2-38c　　　　　　图2-38d

2. 形成邻接关系。

- 将未预备的#21可摘代模放回牙列模型中，并在邻牙上标记颊面接触区的位置（图2-39a）。而后，将蜡型放回牙列模型

- 添加蜡锥，将蜡型和邻牙上的标记连接起来（图2-39b）。继续加蜡，直到蜡锥与标记牢固接触。在蜡完全冷却之前，不要将蜡型从牙列模型中取出。远离接触区部位多余的蜡可以在步骤3中雕刻清除

2. Establish proximal contacts.

- Replace the unprepared tooth #21 in the dentoform to mark the location of the proximal contacts on the buccal surface of the adjacent teeth (Fig 2-39a). Then return the wax-up to the dentoform.

- Add wax cones to connect your wax up with the marks on the adjacent teeth (Fig 2-39b). Continue adding wax until the cones make firm contact with the marks. Do not remove the tooth from the dentoform until the wax cools completely. Excess wax away from the location of the contact can be carved in step 3.

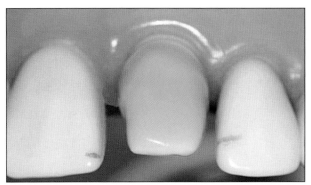
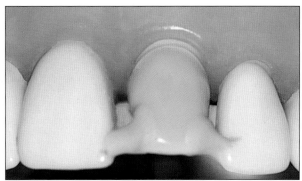

图2-39a　　　　　　　　　　　　　图2-39b

3. 形成邻面接触区。

- 将可摘代模从牙列模型中取出，继续在邻面接触区加蜡至龈方终止线，保持蜡表面相对平坦（图2-40a和b）

- 使用Hollenback雕刻刀，将蜡延伸至覆盖整个邻面（图2-40c）。应注意避免雕刻接触区。邻面应在切龈向和唇舌向的龈方至接触区保持相对平坦

3. Wax the proximal surface.

- Remove the tooth from the dentoform and add wax to join the waxed proximal contact to the gingival finish line, keeping the wax relatively flat (Figs 2-40a and 2-40b).

- Use your Hollenback carver to carve the proximal surfaces flat cervical to the contact (Fig 2-40c). Care should be taken to avoid carving the contact. Proximal surfaces are relatively flat labiolingually and incisocervically between the contact area and the cervical line.

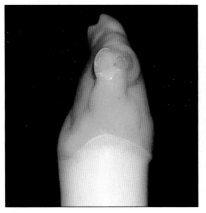
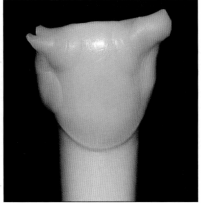
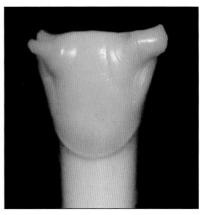

图2-40a   图2-40b   图2-40c

4. 形成切缘。

- 将可摘代模放回牙列模型中，在切缘处加蜡，形成切缘。每次加蜡时都要拖动，从邻牙开始。两颗中切牙的长度应该完全相同；这对美学非常重要。在蜡还未冷却时，轻轻地按压蜡型，使蜡型牙尖和邻牙切缘持平（图2-41a）

- 使用Hollenback雕刻刀进一步调整切缘的长度（图2-41b）。楔状隙可在这一步雕刻或在完成唇面、舌面堆塑后雕刻

- 保持可摘代模在牙列模型中，使用Hollenback雕刻刀雕刻切楔状隙（图2-41c和d）。注意远中切角比近中切角更圆钝，因此远中切楔状隙比近中切楔状隙略大。在堆蜡完成后，进一步调整楔状隙

4. Establish the incisal edge.

- Return the tooth to the dentoform, and add wax to the incisal part of your wax-up to form the incisal edge. The wax is dragged while being added between the proximal ends of the incisal part of the wax-up. Both central incisors should be exactly the same length; this has a major effect on esthetics. With the wax still warm, press the dentoform on the bench to level the incisal edge of your wax-up with the adjacent central incisor (Fig 2-41a).

- The incisal edge length can be further adjusted with the Hollenback carver (Fig 2-41b). Embrasures can be carved following incisal edge adjustment or after the labial or lingual surfaces are waxed.

- With the tooth in the dentoform, carve the incisal embrasures with the Hollenback carver (Figs 2-41c and 2-41d). Remember that the disto-incisal angle is more round than the mesio-incisal angle and that the disto-incisal embrasure is slightly larger than the mesio-incisal embrasure. Further adjustment of the embrasures is done after finishing the wax-up.

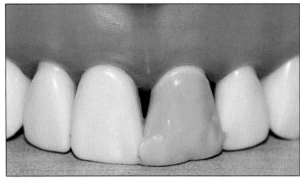
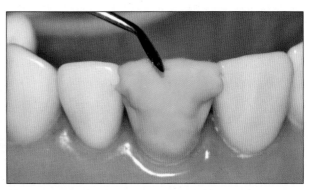

图2-41a   图2-41b

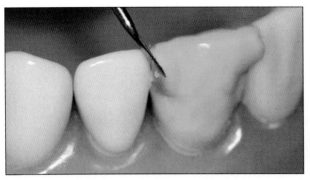

图2-41c

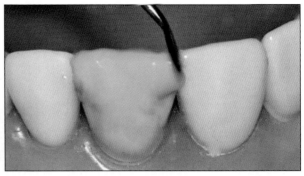

图2-41d

5. 堆塑唇面。

- 保持可摘代模在牙列模型中，在唇面加蜡，完成唇面轮廓（图2-42a）。在颈1/3和唇侧线角处添加更多的蜡

- 唇面塑形。使用超细黑色记号笔粗略标出唇面外形高点和过渡线角的位置。上颌中切牙在牙齿中线的近中和远中有两条浅的唇发育沟。这些都可以从切面观上清楚地看到。标记与相邻中切牙相同的发育沟位置（图2-42b）

- 将可摘代模从牙列模型中取出，在标记区之内雕刻，保持标记位置的线角和外形高点。在完成雕刻后，使用Hollenback雕刻刀轻轻地擦掉黑色标记线。使用Hollenback雕刻刀雕刻唇面大部分。使用盘-爪状雕刻刀的大工作尖（使用盘状部分）从颈1/3到切嵴来雕刻发育沟（图2-42c）。轻柔雕刻，以避免在蜡型上留下无法抛光的凹痕（图2-42d）

5. Wax the labial surface.

- With the tooth in the dentoform, add a layer of wax to the labial surface to complete the labial contour (Fig 2-42a). Apply more wax at the cervical third and the labial line angles.

- Labial surface carving. With the ultrafine-point black marker, roughly mark the locations of the labial height of contour and the transitional line angles. The maxillary central incisors have two shallow labial developmental depressions mesial and distal to the midline of the tooth. These can clearly be seen from an incisal view. Mark the location of these depressions identical to those on the adjacent central incisor (Fig 2-42b).

- Remove the tooth from the dentoform and carve between the marks and outside the marks, keeping the line angles and the height of contour at the marked locations. The black marks can be gently erased with the Hollenback carver after you are done carving. The labial surface is mostly carved with the Hollenback carver. The developmental depressions can be carved with the large discoid-cleoid carver (using the discoid part) from the cervical third toward the incisal ridge (Fig 2-42c). Carving should be gentle to avoid leaving gouges in the tooth that cannot be polished (Fig 2-42d).

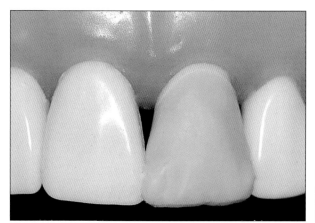

图2-42a

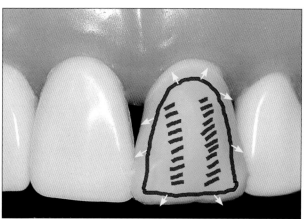

图2-42b　雕刻方向（黄色箭头）和发育沟（黑色线阴影）。参照相邻中切牙雕刻

The direction of carving *(yellow arrows)* and developmental depressions *(black shading)*. These should be carved similar to those on the adjacent central incisor.

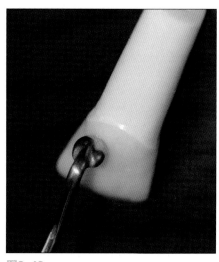

图2-42c

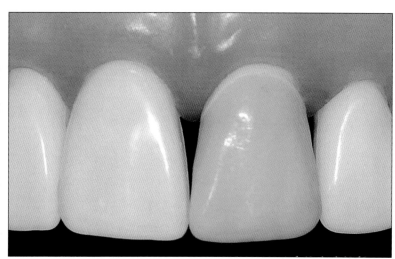

图2-42d　唇面雕刻完成

Labial surface after carving.

6. 堆塑舌面。

- 舌面加一层蜡，完成舌面轮廓。在颈1/3处添加更多的蜡，形成舌隆突。在近中边界和远中边界添加更多的蜡，形成近中边缘嵴和远中边缘嵴（图2-43a）

- 堆塑舌面。使用超细黑色记号笔标记舌窝边界（模仿相邻中切牙）（图2-43b）。将可摘代模从牙列模型中取出，使用盘-爪状雕刻刀的大工作尖雕刻舌窝（图2-43c）。在雕刻舌窝后所有周边的凸起（边缘嵴、舌隆突、切嵴）可以通过最小限度地修形和抛光来强调（图2-43d）

6. Wax the lingual surface.

- Add a layer of wax to the lingual surface to complete the lingual contour. Apply more wax at the cervical third to form the cingulum. Apply more wax at the mesial and distal boundaries to form the marginal ridges (Fig 2-43a).

- Lingual surface carving. Mark the lingual fossa boundaries with the ultrafine-point black marker (mimic the adjacent central incisor) (Fig 2-43b). With the tooth out of the dentoform, carve the lingual fossa with the large discoid-cleoid carver (Fig 2-43c). All the surrounding elevations (marginal ridges, cingulum, and incisal ridge) can be easily emphasized with minimal contouring and polishing after carving the lingual fossa (Fig 2-43d).

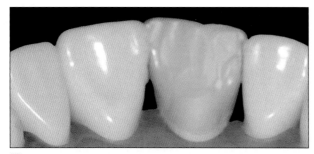

图2-43a

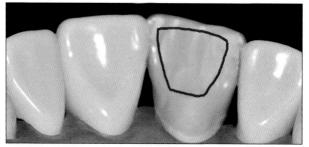

图2-43b

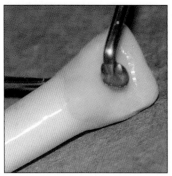

图2-43c

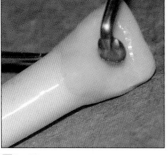

图2-43d

7. 完成最终的雕刻和修形。
- 从不同角度检查线角、点角、楔状隙、邻面接触区、切缘、舌面解剖结构、外形高点和终止线。根据需要进行加蜡和雕刻，来最终实现蜡型形态与相邻中切牙一致及与牙列中其余牙齿和谐（图2-44）

7. Complete final carving and contouring.
- Line angles, point angles, embrasures, proximal contacts, incisal edge, lingual anatomy, heights of contour, and finish line are all checked from different views. Wax addition and carving is done as needed to achieve a final wax-up that is consistent with the adjacent central incisor and harmonious with the rest of the dentition (Fig 2-44).

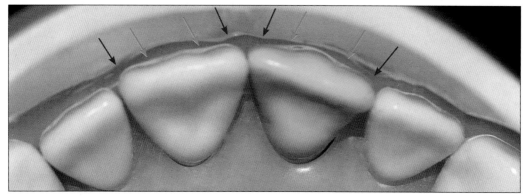

图2-44a 最好从切面观来观察唇侧线角（红色箭头）和唇发育沟（绿色箭头），位置和轮廓应与相邻中切牙一致

The labial line angles *(red arrows)* and the labial developmental depressions *(green arrows)* are best visualized from the incisal view and should conform in position and contour with those of the adjacent central incisor.

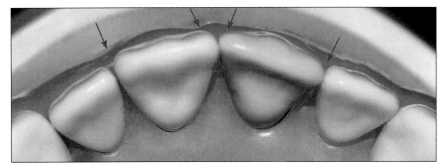

图2-44b　最好从切面观来观察点角（箭头所示），位置和轮廓应与相邻中切牙一致

The point angles *(arrows)* are best visualized from the incisal view and should conform in position and contour to those of the adjacent central incisor.

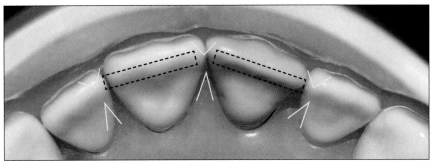

图2-44c　从切面观来观察唇楔状隙和舌楔状隙（黄色标记），位置和轮廓应与相邻中切牙一致。切缘（虚线框）的宽度和厚度应与相邻中切牙一致

The labial and lingual embrasures *(in yellow)* are visualized from the incisal view and should match the contralateral embrasures in size and location. The width and thickness of the incisal edge *(dotted box)* should conform to that of the adjacent central incisor

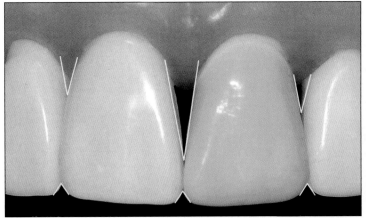

图2-44d　从唇面观或舌面观来观察切楔状隙和颈邻间隙（黄色标记）。远中切楔状隙比近中切楔状隙略大，远中切角更圆钝。和未预备的#21可摘代模比对切楔状隙的大小

Incisal and cervical embrasures *(in yellow)* are visualized from labial or lingual views. The disto-incisal embrasure is slightly larger than the mesio-incisal embrasure given the more rounded disto-incisal point angle. You can compare the mesio-incisal embrasure with the unprepared tooth #21 to match the size of the embrasure accurately.

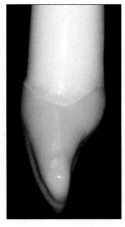

图2-44e

将蜡型从牙列模型中取出，确认邻牙与蜡型之间的邻接面是平滑过渡的。和未预备的#21可摘代模比对唇舌径的大小

Out of the dentoform, verify that the transition from the unprepared tooth to the wax is smooth. Hold the unprepared tooth #21 adjacent to your wax-up and compare contours.

8. 完成最终的平整和抛光。

- 使用雕刻刀修平表面，再使用尼龙布轻轻抛光。这应该会让蜡型看起来更漂亮。应避免长时间地打磨，因为这会改变牙体的结构。为了避免破坏蜡型，抛光时勿过度加压。使用注射器吹气或刷子清除蜡型和牙列模型上多余的蜡屑（图2-45）

8. Complete final smoothing and polishing.

- Plane the surface with a carver and buff lightly with a nylon stocking. This should give your wax-up a nice polished appearance. Avoid lengthy polishing, as it may change the tooth anatomy, and use only gentle pressure to avoid breaking your wax-up. Remove wax flakes on your wax-up and the dentoform using the airway syringe or a brush (Fig 2-45).

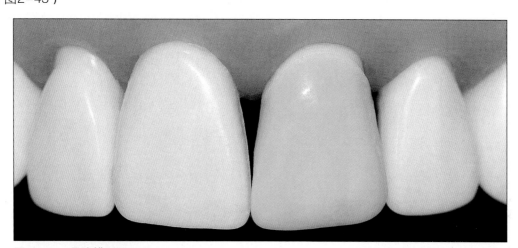

图2-45a 最终蜡型唇面观
Labial view of final wax-up.

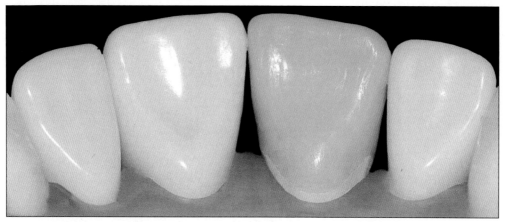

图2-45b 最终蜡型舌面观
Lingual view of final wax-up.

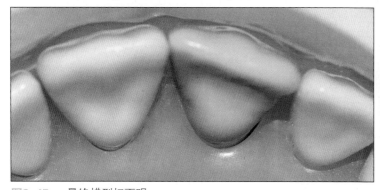

图2-45c 最终蜡型切面观
Incisal view of final wax-up.

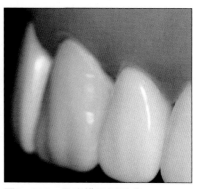

图2-45d 最终蜡型邻面观
Proximal view of final wax-up.

堆塑尖牙蜡型
Waxing Canines

上颌尖牙全冠蜡型堆塑的形态和标准[6-7]

唇面观

从唇面观可以观察到（图3-1a）：

- 外形呈五边形
- 一个牙尖，远中牙尖嵴比近中牙尖嵴长（牙尖顶偏近中）
- 牙尖嵴形态可能是平缓的或略凹的，其长度和轮廓与对侧同名牙一致
- 唇轴嵴是从牙尖顶延伸至唇面外形高点的隆起
- 唇轴嵴的近中和远中有两条浅的纵向发育沟
- 近中接触区位于切1/3和中1/3交界处
- 远中接触区位于中1/3的中心
- 切楔状隙和颈邻间隙的大小、位置与对侧同名牙一致
- 切颈径（即牙冠长度）与对侧同名牙一致

Morphology and Criteria for Maxillary Canine Full-Crown Wax-Up[6,7]

Labial view

The following can be observed in the labial view (Fig 3-1a):

- Pentagonal outline.
- One cusp. The distal cusp ridge is longer than the mesial cusp ridge (the cusp tip is positioned mesially).
- Cusp ridges may be flat or slightly concave and are consistent in length and contour with those of the contralateral tooth.
- Labial ridge is a convex elevation that extends from the cusp tip to the labial height of contour.
- Two shallow longitudinal depressions exist mesial and distal to the labial ridge.
- Mesial contact area at the junction of incisal and middle thirds of the crown.
- Distal contact area at the center of the middle third of the crown.
- Incisal and cervical embrasures consistent in size and location with those of the contralateral canine.
- Incisocervical dimension (ie, length of the tooth) consistent with the contralateral canine.

舌面观

从舌面观可以观察到（图3-1b）：

- 牙冠向舌侧缩窄
- 舌面解剖学特征较为显著
- 舌隆突在所有前牙中最大，大小和轮廓与对侧同名牙一致
- 边缘嵴明显，与邻牙边缘嵴处于同一水平面
- 舌轴嵴从舌隆突近切缘侧延伸至牙尖顶，与对侧同名牙一致
- 舌轴嵴将舌窝分为近中舌窝和远中舌窝，其深度和宽度与对侧同名牙一致且对称

Lingual view

The following can be observed in the lingual view (Fig 3-1b):

- Crown tapers lingually.
- Well-developed lingual anatomy.
- Largest cingulum of all anterior teeth and consistent with that of the contralateral canine in size and contour.
- Marginal ridges strongly developed and at the same level as the adjacent marginal ridges.
- Lingual ridge extends from the incisal portion of the cingulum to the cusp tip and is consistent with that of the contralateral canine.
- Lingual ridge divides the lingual fossa into mesial and distal lingual fossae, which are distinct and consistent in depth and width with those of the contralateral canine.

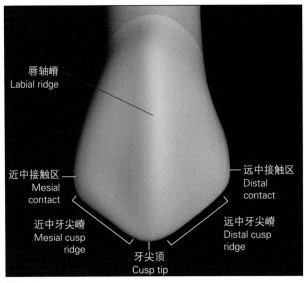

图3-1a

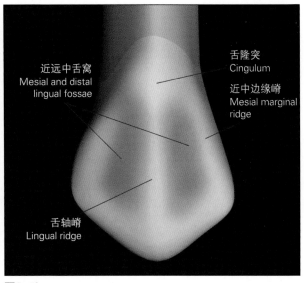

图3-1b

邻面观

从邻面观可以观察到（图3-1c和d）：

- 外形呈三角形
- 唇面轮廓的突度和平滑度与对侧同名牙一致
- 舌面轮廓凸起部分位于颈1/3，凹陷部分位于中1/3和切1/3交界处，并与对侧同名牙一致
- 牙尖顶略偏于牙根唇舌径等分线的唇侧
- 唇舌径与对侧同名牙一致

Proximal view

The following can be observed in the proximal views (Figs 3-1c and 3-1d):

- Triangular outline.
- Labial outline convex and smooth over its entire length and consistent with the contralateral canine.
- Lingual outline convex in the cervical third, concave over the middle and incisal thirds, and consistent with the contralateral canine.
- Cusp tip slightly labial to a line bisecting the root labiolingually.
- Faciolingual dimension of the tooth consistent with that of the contralateral canine.

切面观

从切面观可以观察到（图3-1e）：

- 外形呈钻石形
- 唇舌径比近远中径大
- 牙尖顶位于牙体长轴偏唇侧和近中侧
- 唇面突度比切牙更大
- 唇尖突出，与对侧同名牙一致
- 所有点角及线角的位置和轮廓与对侧同名牙一致
- 唇楔状隙和舌楔状隙的大小、位置与对侧同名牙一致，舌楔状隙较宽

Incisal view

The following can be observed in the incisal view (Fig 3-1e):

- Diamond outline.
- Labiolingual dimension greater than mesiodistal dimension.
- Tip of the cusp labial and mesial to the long axis of the root.
- Labial surface more convex than that of the incisors.
- Labial cusp prominent and consistent with the contralateral canine.
- All point angles and line angles consistent in position and contour with those of the contralateral canine.
- Labial and lingual embrasures consistent in size and location with the contralateral canine, and the lingual embrasures are wider.

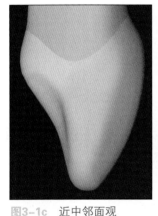

图3-1c 近中邻面观
Mesial view.

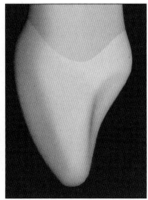

图3-1d 远中邻面观
Distal view.

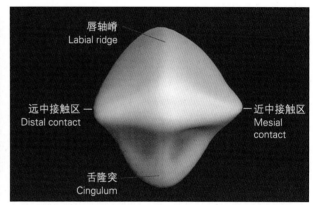

图3-1e

#23全冠蜡型堆塑步骤

尖牙标志着口腔前牙和后牙之间的过渡，并且位于牙弓转折处（图3-2）。制作尖牙蜡型是一项非常重要的训练。在本章中学习如何成形牙尖，将为接下来制作前磨牙和磨牙的蜡型打基础。从牙列模型上取出#23开始，这样可以放置预备好的可摘代模。

Waxing Steps for Tooth #23 Full-Crown Wax-Up

Canines mark the transition between anterior and posterior teeth of the mouth and are located where the arch curves (Fig 3-2). Waxing canines is a very important exercise. You will learn how to form cusps in this exercise, which will prepare you to wax the multicusped premolars and molars in the following chapters. Start by unscrewing tooth #23 from your dentoform so you can place the prepared tooth peg.

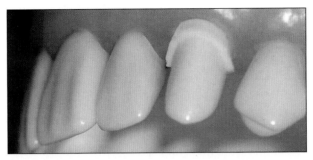

图3-2

1. 形成初始蜡层。

- 手握可摘代模，开始在可摘代模的牙体预备区加蜡（图3-3a和b）。因为尖牙比切牙大，所以要涂一层较厚的初始蜡层。蜡层厚度均匀，不留空隙

- 延长蜡层超过终止线，以确保蜡层边缘没有缺陷（图3-3c）

- 使用Hollenback雕刻刀雕刻蜡型，使之与终止线平齐且轮廓合适，以实现与可摘代模的平滑过渡

1. Establish initial layer of wax.

- With the tooth peg in your hand, start adding wax to cover the prepared area of the tooth peg (Figs 3-3a and 3-3b). A thicker initial layer of wax is applied, given that canines are larger than incisors. The wax should have an even thickness and no voids.

- Extend the wax past the finish line. This is done to ensure that the wax is not deficient at the margin (Fig 3-3c).

- Use the Hollenback carver to carve the wax flush with the finish line and with the proper contour to achieve a smooth transition with the tooth peg.

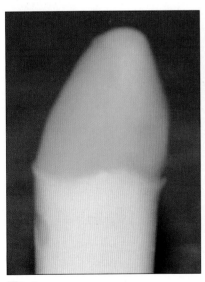
图3-3a

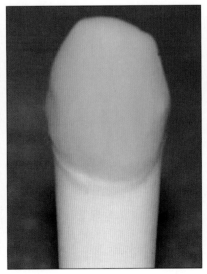
图3-3b

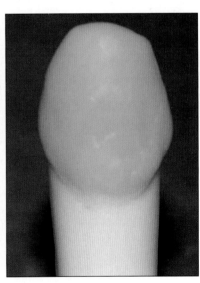
图3-3c

2. 形成邻接关系。

- 标记邻牙邻面接触区的位置（图3-4a）。而后将蜡型放回牙列模型。远中接触区位于#22的中1/3，近中接触区位于#24的𬌗1/3和中1/3交界处。两个邻面接触区都位于唇舌径/颊舌径中央偏唇/颊侧。复制对侧同名牙的接触区位置

2. Establish proximal contacts.

- Mark the location for the proximal contacts on the adjacent teeth (Fig 3-4a), then return the wax-up to the dentoform. The distal contact on tooth #22 is at the middle third, and the mesial contact on #24 is at the junction of occlusal and middle thirds. Both contacts are facial to the center of the crown faciolingually. Duplicate the contact location on the conralateral side.

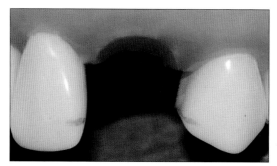

图3-4a

- 添加蜡锥，将蜡型和邻牙上的标记连接起来。继续加蜡，直到蜡锥与标记牢固接触（图3-4b和c）。无论何时对邻面接触区堆蜡时，都应在近唇/颊侧的表面加蜡，因为所有邻面接触区都位于唇舌径/颊舌径中央偏唇/颊侧。蜡锥应与邻牙外形高点（即最大突度）连接。在蜡完全冷却之前，不要将蜡型从牙列模型中取出。远离接触区部位多余的蜡可以在步骤3中雕刻清除

- Add wax cones to connect your wax up with the marks on the adjacent teeth. Continue adding wax until the cones make firm contact with the marks (Figs 3-4b and 3-4c). Whenever proximal contacts are waxed, the wax should always be added on the facial surface because all proximal contacts are facial to the center of the crown faciolingually. The wax cones should contact the adjacent teeth at their height of contour (ie, maximum convexity). Do not remove the tooth from the dentoform until the wax cools completely. Excess wax away from the location of the contact can be carved in step 3.

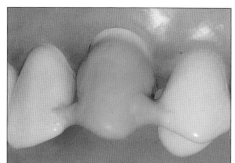

图3-4b 唇面观
Labial view.

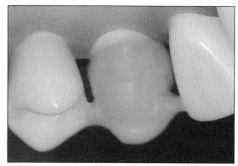

图3-4c 舌面观
Lingual view.

3. 形成邻面接触区。

- 将可摘代模从牙列模型中取出，继续在邻面接触区加蜡至龈方终止线，保持蜡表面相对平坦（图3-5a）。这一步需使用更多的蜡，因为与堆塑切牙相比，尖牙较大并且唇舌径也较大

- 使用Hollenback雕刻刀雕刻邻面，由颈缘至邻面接触区修平表面（图3-5b）

- 将可摘代模放回牙列模型中，邻面接触区应形成良好封闭且位置正确，邻面应在切龈向和唇舌向的龈方至接触区保持平坦（图3-5c和d）

3. Waxing the proximal surface.

- Remove the tooth from the dentoform, and add wax to join the waxed proximal contact to the gingival finish line, keeping the wax relatively flat (Fig 3-5a). More wax is applied at this step when compared with waxing incisors because the canine is a larger tooth and has a larger labiolingual dimension.

- Use the Hollenback carver to carve the proximal surfaces flat cervical to the contact (Fig 3-5b).

- When the tooth is returned to the dentoform, the proximal contact should be properly closed and at the right location, and the proximal surface should be flat cervical to the contact in the incisogingival and labiolingual directions (Figs 3-5c and 3-5d).

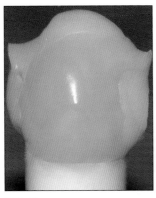
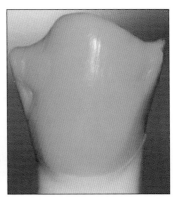

图3-5a　　　　　　图3-5b

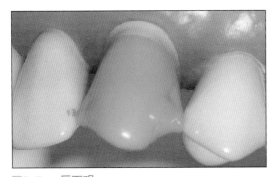

图3-5c　唇面观
Labial view.

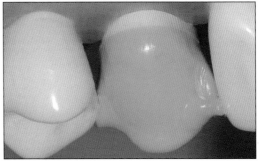

图3-5d　舌面观
Lingual view.

4. 形成牙尖。

- 定位牙尖顶。把未预备的#23可摘代模放回牙列模型中，从切面观和唇面观来观察尖牙牙尖顶的位置，以便形象化地确定蜡型牙尖顶位置（图3-6）。所有的后牙颊尖牙尖顶都处于同一平面，上颌尖牙牙尖应比上颌第一前磨牙的颊尖略长。上颌尖牙牙尖顶偏近中

4. Establish the cusp.

- Locating the cusp tip. Return the unprepared tooth #23 to the dentoform and notice the location of the cusp tip of the canine from the incisal and labial views in order to visualize and locate the wax-up cusp tip (Fig 3-6). All the buccal cusp tips of posterior teeth occur on the same plane. The cusp of the canine should be slightly longer than the buccal cusp of the maxillary first premolar. The cusp tip of the maxillary canine is positioned toward the mesial.

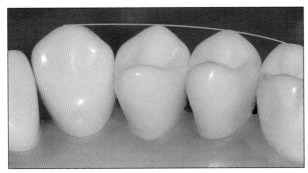

图3-6a

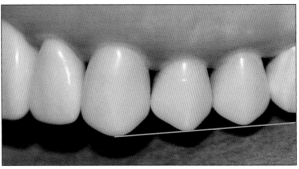

图3-6b

- 堆塑牙尖顶。在牙尖顶的位置堆一个蜡锥（图3-7a）。蜡锥应比上颌第一前磨牙颊尖牙尖顶高

- 确定牙尖高度。在蜡还未冷却时，轻轻地按压蜡型，使蜡型牙尖和对侧同名牙牙尖同时接触工作台平面（图3-7b）。使尖牙蜡型的牙尖变平，高度与对侧同名牙牙尖一致（图3-7c和d）。在最终的雕刻和修形的步骤中，进一步调整牙尖顶的位置/高度

- 堆塑牙尖嵴。为了形成牙尖嵴，添加蜡将相邻牙切/𬌗面与蜡型牙尖顶连接起来（图3-7e和f）。每次加蜡时都要拖动，从邻牙开始，到牙尖顶结束。这项操作不应该干扰原有牙尖顶的高度。通常需要添加1~2层蜡来完成牙尖嵴的堆塑

- 在这一步或唇面堆蜡后，使用Hollenback雕刻刀仔细地调整牙尖嵴（图3-7g）。目标是复制对侧同名牙的高度和轮廓，保持牙尖顶偏近中。避免牙尖过短。如果需要，可在最终的雕刻步骤时进一步修整轮廓。楔状隙可在这一步雕刻或在完成堆塑唇面、舌面后雕刻

- Waxing the cusp tip. Add a wax cone where the cusp tip should be located (Fig 3-7a). The wax cone should be higher than the maxillary first premolar cusp tip.

- Establishing the cusp height. With the wax still warm, gently press your dentoform on the bench so that the contralateral canine and your wax-up are both touching the bench (Fig 3-7b). This will level your wax up of no. 11 with the contralateral canine (Figs 3-7c and 3-7d). Further adjustment of the cusp tip location/height can be done during final carving and contouring of the wax-up.

- Waxing the cusp ridges. To form the cusp ridges, add wax to connect the incisal/occlusal part of the proximal surfaces of the adjacent teeth to the cusp tip (Figs 3-7e and 3-7f). Each wax increment is dragged, starting at the adjacent tooth and ending at the cusp tip. This should *not* interfere with the cusp height you already achieved. Usually one or two increments of wax are needed to complete the ridges.

- Adjustment of the cusp ridges is done carefully with the Hollenback carver at this step or after waxing the labial surface (Fig 3-7g). The goal is to duplicate the height and contour of the cusp ridges of the contralateral canine, keeping the cusp tip offset to the mesial. Avoid overshortening the cusp. Further contouring can be done in the final carving step, if needed. Embrasures can be carved at this step or after the labial or lingual surfaces are waxed.

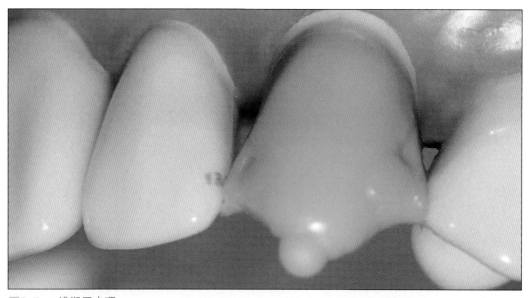

图3-7a 堆塑牙尖顶
Waxing the cusp tip.

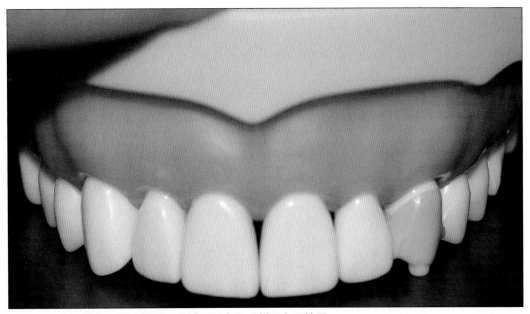

图3-7b　在工作台上按压蜡型，使蜡型牙尖和对侧同名牙持平
Finger press the dentoform on the bench to level your wax-up with the contralateral canine.

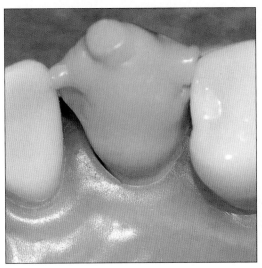

图3-7c　殆面观
Occlusal view.

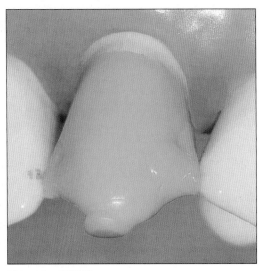

图3-7d　唇面观
Labial view.

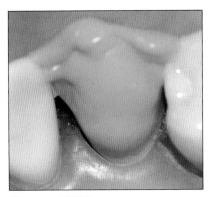

图3-7e　殆面观
Occlusal view.

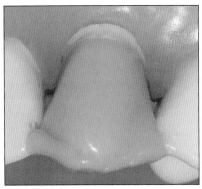

图3-7f　唇面观
Labial view.

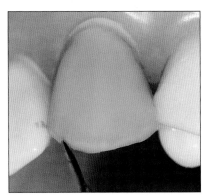

图3-7g

5. 堆塑唇面。

- 在唇面加蜡，完成唇面轮廓。在颈1/3处添加更多的蜡，形成外形高点。然后通过连接近中边界、远中边界和唇面外形高点形成相应的线角。通过连接唇面外形高点近切缘部分到牙尖顶形成唇轴嵴。与切牙相比，上颌尖牙的隆起更明显。保持可摘代模在牙列模型中，添加唇面轮廓，以实现精确定位。可以在对侧同名牙上画出牙面和唇轴嵴来想象这些解剖标志的位置，并把它们精确复制在蜡型上（图3-8a和b）

- 保持可摘代模在牙列模型中，使用Hollenback雕刻刀雕刻切楔状隙（图3-8c~e）。远中切楔状隙比近中切楔状隙略大，因为远中切角比近中切角更圆钝，并且远中邻接位置比近中更靠近颈部。模仿对侧同名牙楔状隙形态。在最终的雕刻和修形步骤中，可以通过加蜡或雕刻点角来进一步调整楔状隙的大小

- 最后添加一层蜡，填充线角、唇轴嵴和外形高点之间的空间（图3-8f）

- 唇面塑形。将可摘代模从牙列模型中取出，标记唇轴嵴、唇侧线角和外形高点的位置（图3-8g）。使用Hollenback雕刻刀来雕刻和精修标记之间的蜡，保持蜡型轮廓位置适当（图3-8h）

5. Wax the labial surface.

- Add wax to the labial surface to complete the labial contour. More wax is applied at the cervical third to form the height of contour. The line angles are then waxed by joining the mesial and distal ends of the labial height of contour to the corresponding cusp ridges. The labial ridge is created by connecting the incisal part of the labial height of contour to the cusp tip. These elevations are more prominent on the maxillary canine compared with the incisors. The contours are added with the tooth in the dentoform for precise localization. You may draw the face of the tooth and the labial ridge on the contralateral canine to visualize the location of these landmarks and duplicate them precisely on your wax-up (Figs 3-8a and 3-8b).

- With the tooth in the dentoform, carve the incisal embrasures with the Hollenback carver (Figs 3-8c to 3-8e). The disto-incisal embrasure is slightly larger than the mesio-incisal embrasure, because the disto-incisal angle is more round than the mesio-incisal angle and the distal contact is more cervical than the mesial contact. Mimic the embrasures on the contralateral canine. The size of the embrasures can be further adjusted in the final carving and contouring step by wax addition or carving at the point angles.

- Add a final layer of wax to fill in the spaces between the line angles, labial ridge, and height of contour (Figs 3-8f).

- Carving the labial surface. With the tooth out of the dentoform, mark the labial ridge, labial line angles, and height of contour (Fig 3-8g). Use the Hollenback carver to carve and refine the wax between and away from the marks, keeping your contours at the proper location (Fig 3-8h).

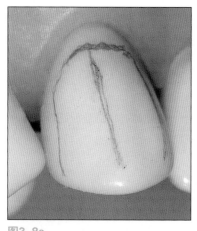

图3-8a

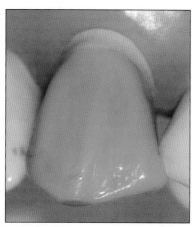

图3-8b

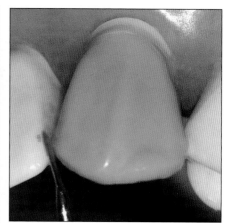

图3-8c

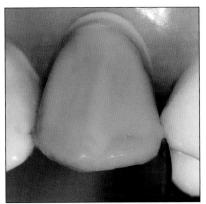

图3-8d

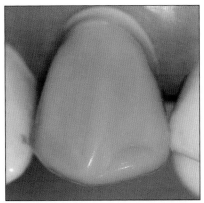

图3-8e

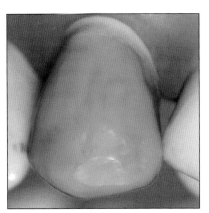

图3-8f

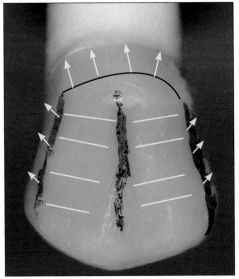

图3-8g　轮廓线（黑色线）和轮廓线之间的
　　　　雕刻方向（黄色箭头）
　　　　Contours (black lines) and the direction
　　　　of the carving (yellow arrows) between
　　　　contours.

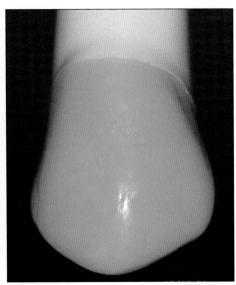

图3-8h

6. 堆塑舌面。

- 舌面加一层蜡，完成舌面轮廓。然后使用更多的蜡来形成上颌尖牙巨大的舌隆突。通过在牙尖顶和舌隆突间拖动加蜡，形成舌轴嵴。通过将舌隆突近中边界和远中边界与相应的牙尖嵴相连，继续堆塑边缘嵴。这一步将完成舌窝的边界。可以在对侧同名牙上画出这些解剖标志来想象它们的位置，并把其精确复制在蜡型上（图3-9a和b）

- 加蜡填充舌窝，完成舌面轮廓（图3-9c；这是舌面唯一凹陷的部分）

6. Wax the lingual surface.

- Add a layer of wax to the lingual surface to complete the lingual contour. More wax is then applied to form the bulky cingulum of the maxillary canine. The lingual ridge is then formed by dragging wax between the cusp tip and incisal part of the cingulum. Proceed to create the marginal ridges by joining the mesial and distal boundaries of the cingulum to the corresponding cusp ridges. This will complete the boundaries of the lingual fossae. You may draw these landmarks on the contralateral canine to visualize their location and duplicate them precisely on your wax-up (Figs 3-9a and 3-9b).

- Add wax to fill in the lingual fossae to complete the lingual contour (Fig 3-9c; This is the only part of the lingual surface that may be deficient at this point).

- 雕刻舌面。舌面雕刻和塑形可在牙列模型外完成（图3-9d），使用Hollenback雕刻刀雕刻舌隆突和边缘嵴，使用盘-爪状雕刻刀的小工作尖雕刻舌窝。尖牙近中边缘嵴要修整到和相邻切牙远中边缘嵴同一水平

- Carving the lingual surface. The lingual surface may be carved and contoured with the tooth outside the dentoform (Fig 3-9d), using the Hollenback carver for the cingulum and marginal ridges and using the discoid part of the small discoid-cleoid carver to carve the lingual fossae. The mesial marginal ridge is carved to the level of the distal marginal ridge of the lateral incisor.

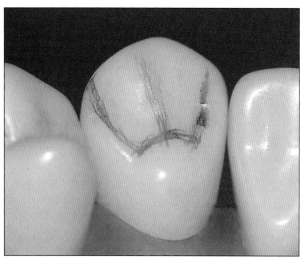

图3-9a

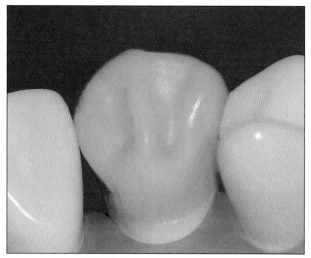

图3-9b

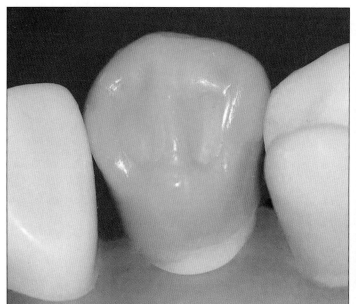

图3-9c　加蜡填充舌窝后的舌面
Lingual surface after filling the fossae with wax.

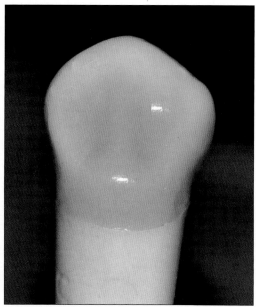

图3-9d　雕刻后的舌面
Lingual surface after carving.

7. 完成最终的雕刻和修形。

• 从不同角度检查线角、点角、楔状隙、邻面接触区、牙尖嵴、舌面解剖结构、外形高点和终止线（图3-10）。根据需要进行加蜡和雕刻，来最终实现蜡型形态与对侧同名牙一致、与邻牙和谐

7. Complete final carving and contouring.

• Line angles, point angles, embrasures, proximal contacts, cusp ridges, lingual anatomy, heights of contour, and finish line are all checked from different views (Fig 3-10). Wax addition and carving is done as needed to achieve a final wax-up that is consistent with the contralateral canine and harmonious with the adjacent teeth.

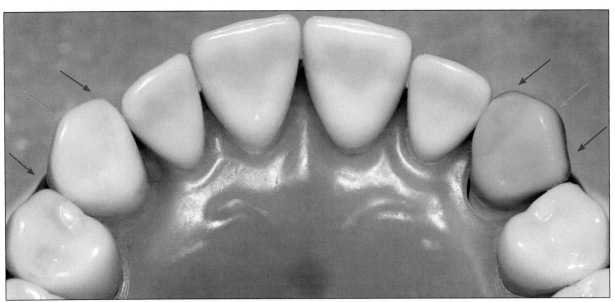

图3-10a　最好从切面观来观察唇侧线角（红色箭头）和唇轴嵴（绿色箭头），位置和轮廓应与对侧同名牙一致
The labial line angles *(red arrows)* and labial ridges *(green arrow)* are best visualized from the incisal view and should conform in position and contour with those of the contralateral canine.

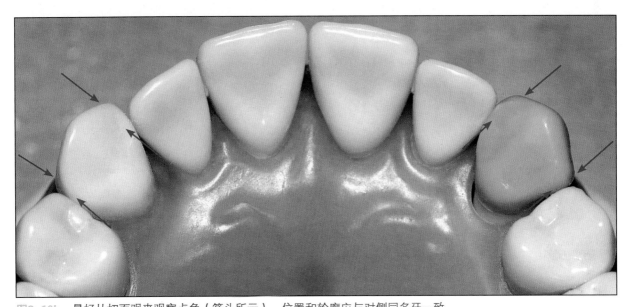

图3-10b　最好从切面观来观察点角（箭头所示），位置和轮廓应与对侧同名牙一致
The point angles *(arrows)* are best visualized from the incisal view and should conform in position and contour to those of the contralateral canine.

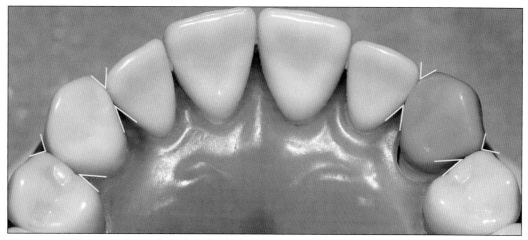

图3-10c 从切面观来观察唇楔状隙和舌楔状隙（黄色标记），大小、位置应与对侧楔状隙一致

The labial and lingual embrasures *(in yellow)* are visualized from the incisal view and should match the contralateral embrasures in size and location.

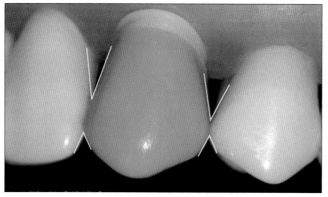

图3-10d 从唇面观或舌面观来观察切楔状隙和颈邻间隙（黄色标记）。远中切楔状隙比近中切楔状隙略大，远中切角更圆钝

Incisal and cervical embrasures *(in yellow)* are visualized from a labial or lingual view. The disto-incisal embrasure is slightly larger than the mesio-incisal embrasure given the more rounded disto-incisal point angle.

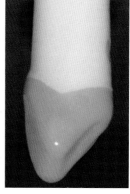

图3-10e

将蜡型从牙列模型中取出，确认邻牙与蜡型之间的邻接面是平滑过渡的。和未预备的#23可摘代模比对唇舌径的大小

Remove the wax-up from the dentoform and verify that the transition from the un-prepared tooth to the wax is smooth. Compare your labio-lingual dimension to the un-prepared tooth #23.

8. 完成最终的平整和抛光。

• 使用雕刻刀修平表面，再使用尼龙布轻轻抛光。这应该会让蜡型看起来更漂亮（图3-11）。应避免长时间地打磨，因为这会改变牙体的结构。为了避免破坏蜡型，抛光时勿过度加压。使用注射器吹气或刷子清除蜡型和牙列模型上多余的蜡屑

8. Complete the final smoothing and polishing.
   • Plane the surface with a carver and buff lightly with a nylon stocking. This should give your wax-up a nice polished appearance (Fig 3-11). Avoid lengthy polishing as it may change the tooth anatomy. Use only gentle pressure to avoid breaking your wax-up. Remove wax flakes on your wax-up and dentoform using the airway syringe or a brush.

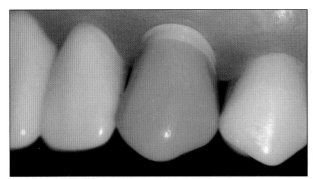

图3-11a 最终蜡型唇面观
Labial view of final wax-up.

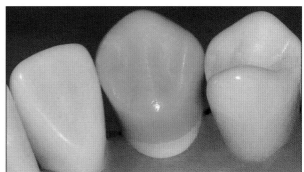

图3-11b 最终蜡型舌面观
Lingual view of final wax-up.

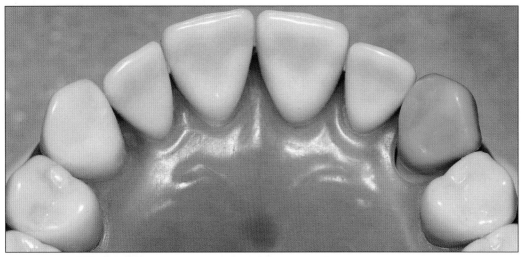

图3-11c 最终蜡型切面观
Incisal view of final wax-up.

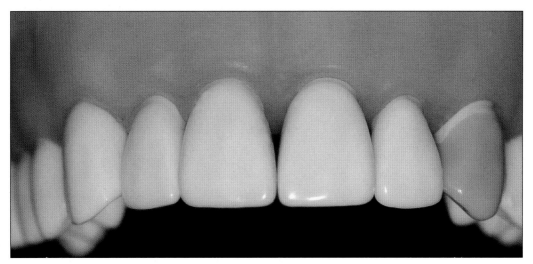

图3-11d 最终蜡型邻面观
Proximal view of final wax-up.

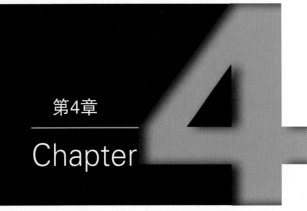

堆塑前磨牙蜡型
Waxing Premolars

上颌第一前磨牙全冠蜡型堆塑的形态和标准[6-7]

颊面观

从颊面观可以观察到（图4-1a）：

- 外形呈五边形
- 颊尖相对较长，与尖牙牙尖相似但略短
- 颊尖的远中牙尖嵴比近中牙尖嵴短（牙尖顶偏远中）
- 颊轴嵴是从颊尖牙尖顶延伸至颊面外形高点的隆起
- 颊轴嵴的近中和远中可以看到两条发育沟
- 颊侧线角突出，且位置和轮廓与对侧同名牙一致
- 颊侧点角突出，且位置和轮廓与对侧同名牙一致
- 近中和远中接触区位于𬌗1/3与中1/3交界处，偏颊侧

Morphology and Criteria for Maxillary First Premolar Full-Crown Wax-Up[6,7]

Buccal view

The following can be observed in the buccal view (Fig 4-1a):

- Geometric outline is pentagonal.
- Buccal cusp relatively long and resembles the cusp of the canine but slightly shorter than the canine cusp.
- Distal cusp ridge of the buccal cusp shorter than the mesial cusp ridge (The cusp tip is positioned distally).
- Buccal ridge is the convex elevation that extends from the buccal cusp tip to the buccal height of contour.
- Two developmental depressions may be seen mesial and distal to the buccal ridge.
- Buccal line angles prominent and conform to those of the contralateral premolar in position and contour.
- Buccal point angles prominent and conform to those of the contralateral premolar in position and contour.
- Mesial and distal contact areas located at the junction of occlusal and middle thirds and toward the buccal.

- 颈邻间隙和拾楔状隙与对侧同名牙一致
- 拾颈径（即牙冠长度）与对侧同名牙一致

舌面观

从舌面观可以观察到（图4-1b）：
- 舌面近远中径比颊面近远中径小（即舌向聚合）
- 舌面外形高点位于中1/3处
- 舌轴嵴是从颈缘线延伸至舌尖牙尖顶的隆起
- 舌尖比颊尖短小
- 舌尖牙尖顶略偏近中
- 有两条凸起的牙尖嵴
- 舌侧线角不如颊侧线角显著
- 舌面在近远向和拾颈向均有凸起

Lingual view

The following can be observed in the lingual view (Fig 4-1b):
- Lingual surface narrower mesiodistally than the buccal surface (ie, lingual convergence).
- Lingual height of contour located in the middle third.
- Lingual ridge is a prominent elevation and extends from the cervical line to the lingual cusp tip.
- Lingual cusp shorter than the buccal cusp.
- Cusp tip of the lingual cusp positioned slightly mesially.
- Both cusp ridges convex.
- Lingual line angles less prominent than the buccal line angles.
- Lingual surface convex mesiodistally and occluso-cervically.

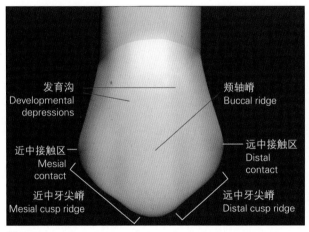

图4-1a

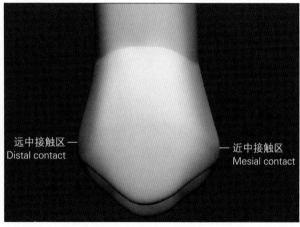

图4-1b

邻面观

从邻面观可以观察到（图4-1c和d）：
- 外形呈梯形
- 舌尖比颊尖短约1mm
- 颊面外形高点位于颈1/3
- 舌面轮廓光滑，凸起，外形高点位于中1/3

Proximal view

The following can be observed in the proximal views (Figs 4-1c and 4-1d):
- Geometric outline is trapezoidal.
- Lingual cusp shorter than the buccal cusp by approximately 1 mm.
- Buccal outline shows the height of contour in the cervical third.
- Lingual outline smooth, convex with the height of contour in the middle third.

- 有发育沟跨过近中边缘嵴，称为近中沟。没有发育沟跨过远中边缘嵴
- 两条隆起的三角嵴斜度较大，呈斜坡状，从牙尖顶延伸至中央沟，在沟底汇合
- 颊舌径与对侧同名牙一致

𬌗面观

从𬌗面观可以观察到（图4-1e）：

- 外形呈六边形
- 𬌗面外形向舌侧缩窄
- 颊尖比舌尖宽且长
- 颊舌径比近远中径大
- 𬌗面形态由突出的颊舌尖、牙尖嵴、三角嵴、边缘嵴、窝（中央窝和两个三角窝）、中央沟和近中沟组成
- 颊尖牙尖顶略偏远中
- 舌尖牙尖顶略偏近中
- 作为中央沟的延续，近中沟跨过近中边缘嵴并延伸至近中面
- 线角及点角的位置和轮廓与对侧同名牙一致
- 舌侧线角不如颊侧线角显著
- 边缘嵴与邻牙的边缘嵴处于同一水平
- 颊楔状隙和舌楔状隙的大小、位置与对侧同名牙一致

- Mesial marginal ridge crossed by a groove called the *mesial marginal developmental groove*. Distal marginal ridge not crossed by a groove.
- Triangular ridges convex and slope from the cusp tips to the central groove where they meet. They are considered quite steep.
- Buccolingual dimension of the tooth consistent with the contralateral premolar.

Occlusal view

The following can be observed in the occlusal view (Fig 4-1e):

- Geometric outline is hexagonal.
- Occlusal outline tapers lingually.
- Buccal cusp wider and longer than the lingual cusp.
- Buccolingual dimension greater than the mesiodistal dimension.
- Occlusal morphology consists of prominent buccal and lingual cusps, cusp ridges, triangular ridges, marginal ridges, occlusal fossae (the central fossa and two triangular fossae), the central developmental groove, and the mesial marginal developmental groove.
- Buccal cusp tip located slightly distal to the midline.
- Lingual cusp tip located slightly mesial to the midline.
- Mesial marginal developmental groove is a continuation of the central groove that crosses the mesial marginal ridge and extends onto the mesial surface.
- Line angles and point angles consistent in position and contour with those of the contralateral tooth.
- Lingual line angles less prominent than the buccal line angles.
- Marginal ridges at the same level as the adjacent marginal ridges.
- Buccal and lingual embrasures consistent in size and location with the contralateral tooth.

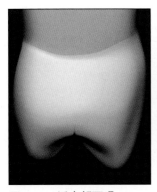

图4-1c 近中邻面观
Mesial view.

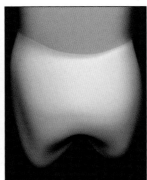

图4-1d 远中邻面观
Distal view.

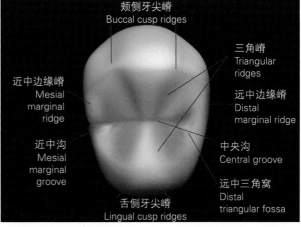

图4-1e

蜡型堆塑入门练习1：#24颊面

本练习主要是在牙列模型外完成的（图4-2）。蜡型堆塑结束后，可将可摘代模放入牙列模型中检查最终轮廓。

1. 确定牙齿预备区域的终止线。请注意，缺失的牙齿结构延伸至颈缘线以下的牙根表面（图4-3）。

Introductory Waxing Exercise 1: Buccal of Tooth #24

This exercise is mainly done outside the dentoform (Fig 4-2). The tooth may be placed in the dentoform to check the final contours after finishing the wax-up.

1. Identify the finish line of the prepared area of the tooth. Notice that the missing tooth structure extends onto the root surface below the cervical line (Fig 4-3).

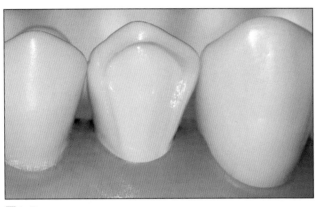

图4-2

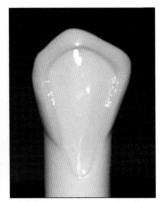

图4-3

2. 使用堆蜡工具，在颊面缺损部位加蜡，直到蜡层覆盖整个预备区（图4-4）。

2. Use wax-addition instruments to start adding wax to the missing buccal surface until the entire prepared area is covered with wax (Fig 4-4).

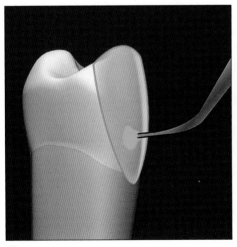

图4-4a

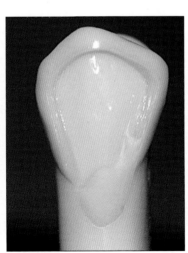

图4-4b

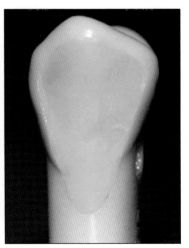

图4-4c

3. 堆塑颊面轮廓：颊轴嵴、线角、外形高点。在颈1/3处加蜡，形成颊面外形高点，相对于颈缘线而言，外形高点突出颊侧颈缘线约0.5mm（图4-5）。拖动蜡滴，通过将外形高点殆方部分的近中边界和远中边界连接到相应的颊侧牙尖嵴来形成颊侧线角。拖动蜡滴，通过将颊面外形高点殆方部分连接到颊尖牙尖顶来形成颊轴嵴。这些特征在上颌第一前磨牙上非常明显，应该与对侧同名牙一致。

4. 清除表面和边缘多余的蜡，将Hollenback雕刻刀部分放在蜡上，部分放在可摘代模上，使蜡面平整光滑（图4-6）。

3. Wax the buccal contours: buccal ridge, line angles, height of contour. Add wax to create the buccal height of contour in the cervical third, which projects about 0.5 mm buccal to the cervical line (Fig 4-5). Form the buccal line angles by dragging wax to connect the mesial and distal sides of the occlusal part of the height of contour to the corresponding buccal cusp ridges. Form the buccal ridge by dragging wax between the occlusal part of the buccal height of contour and the buccal cusp tip. These features are quite prominent on the maxillary first premolar and should be consistent with the contralateral premolar.

4. Carve the excess wax at the margin by resting the Hollenback carver partly on the tooth peg and partly on the wax, then plane and smooth the wax surface (Fig 4-6).

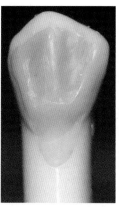 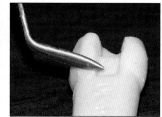

图4-5　　　　　图4-6

5. 使用盘-爪状雕刻刀的小工作尖雕刻近中发育沟、远中发育沟。这样，从殆面观来看，颊面轮廓与对侧同名牙镜像精确一致（图4-7）。

6. 考虑到缺损牙体组织延伸至颈缘线的根方，需要在颊面雕刻颈缘线（图4-8）。这一步可以使用橡子形抛光器。

5. Carve the mesial and distal developmental depressions using the small discoid-cleoid carver, so that, from an occlusal view, the buccal surface is contoured as an exact mirror image of the contralateral first premolar (Fig 4-7).

6. Carve the cervical line on the buccal surface, given that the missing tooth structure extends apical to this line (Fig 4-8). The acorn burnisher can be used for this step.

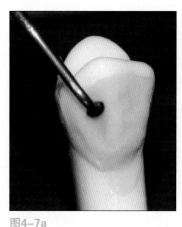 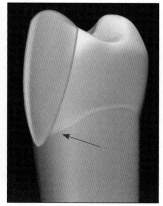

图4-7a　　　　　图4-7b　　　　　图4-8

7. 精修和平整蜡型，然后使用注射器吹气或刷子清除多余的蜡屑。使用尼龙布抛光蜡型（图4-9）。

7. Refine and smooth your wax-up, then brush off excess particles of wax with the airway syringe or a brush. Polish the wax-up with a nylon stocking (Fig 4-9).

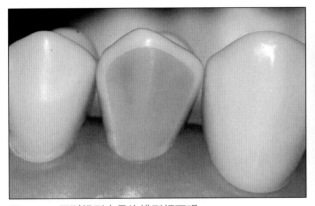
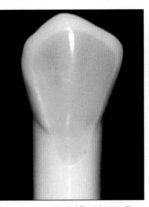
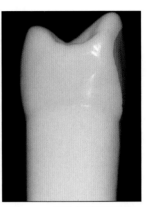

图4-9a　牙列模型中最终蜡型颊面观
Buccal view of final wax-up in the dentoform.

图4-9b　最终蜡型颊面观
Buccal view of final wax-up.

图4-9c　最终蜡型邻面观
Proximal view of final wax-up.

蜡型堆塑入门练习2：#24邻𬌗面

Introductory Waxing Exercise 2: Mesio-Occlusal of Tooth #24

本练习中使用前一次练习所使用的同一个可摘代模。该可摘代模𬌗面及近中面有缺损部分。

1. 注意可摘代模上近中邻𬌗缺损部分的终止线范围（图4-10）。

2. 使用堆蜡工具，在近中面和𬌗面加蜡，形成初始蜡层，直到蜡层覆盖可摘代模所有终止线（图4-11）。

The same tooth peg used in the previous exercise is used in this exercise. The tooth peg has a part of the occlusal and mesial surfaces missing.

1. Notice the extent of your finish line in the mesio-occlusal part of the tooth peg (Fig 4-10).

2. Use your wax-addition instruments to add an initial layer of wax to the missing mesial and occlusal surfaces, covering all of the finish line on the tooth peg (Fig 4-11).

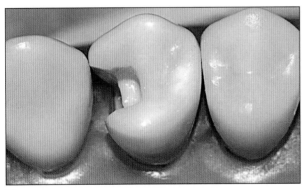
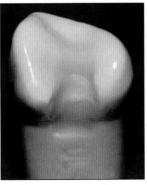
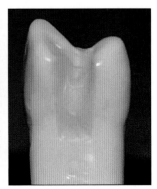

图4-10

图4-11a

图4-11b

3. 将可摘代模放回牙列模型中，并加蜡，形成可摘代模上的近中接触区（图4-12）。

3. Return the tooth to the dentoform, and add wax to complete the mesial contact on the tooth peg (Fig 4-12).

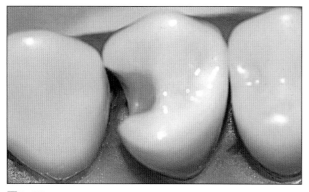

图4-12a

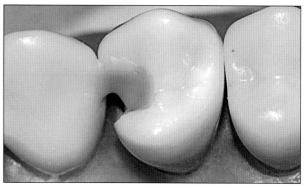

图4-12b

4. 加蜡连接蜡型的近中接触区和可摘代模预备体的舌侧部分，形成近中边缘嵴。然后使用Hollenback雕刻刀修平边缘嵴。边缘嵴可为堆塑近中面和𬌗面提供轮廓，因此通常在堆塑这些表面之前形成边缘嵴（图4-13）。

4. Add wax to create the mesial marginal ridge by connecting the mesial contact of the wax-up with the lingual portion of the prepared tooth peg. Then plane the marginal ridge with the Hollenback carver. The marginal ridge is usually added before waxing the proximal and occlusal surfaces because it provides an outline when waxing those surfaces (Fig 4-13).

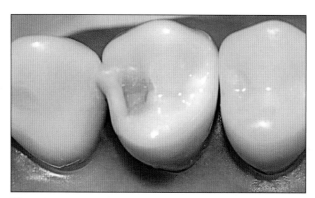

图4-13

5. 堆塑近中面。将可摘代模从牙列模型中取出，并在边缘嵴下方加蜡（图4-14a）。用蜡填充整个表面，保持蜡表面相对平坦（图4-14b）。使用Hollenback雕刻刀雕刻和修平多余的蜡，然后使用橡子形抛光器雕刻颈缘线，颈缘线向𬌗方凸起以便与可摘代模上的颈缘线相连（图4-14c）。

5. Waxing the proximal surface. Remove the tooth from the dentoform and add wax below the marginal ridge (Fig 4-14a). Fill the entire surface with wax, keeping the surface relatively flat (Fig 4-14b). Carve and plane the excess wax with the Hollenback carver, and then carve the cervical line with the acorn burnisher, curving occlusally to continue with the cervical line on your tooth peg (Fig 4-14c).

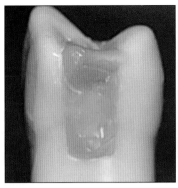
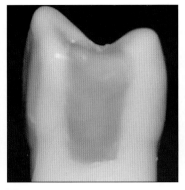
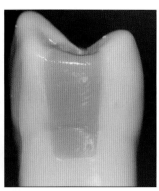

图4-14a　　　　　　　　　　图4-14b　　　　　　　　　　图4-14c

6. 堆塑𬌗面。在𬌗面加蜡，形成三角嵴（图 4-15）。这些三角嵴从牙尖顶向𬌗面中央延伸，并向近中边界和远中边界倾斜，形似一个金字塔。然后使用橡子形抛光器刻出中央沟，中央沟要与可摘代模𬌗面未预备区的中央沟成一直线。

6. Waxing the occlusal surface. Add wax to the occlusal surface to complete the triangular ridges (Fig 4-15). These ridges slope from the cusp tip to the center of the occlusal surface and toward the mesial and distal sides, like a pyramid. Then use the acorn burnisher to carve the central groove, which should be in line with the central groove on the unprepared occlusal surface of the tooth peg.

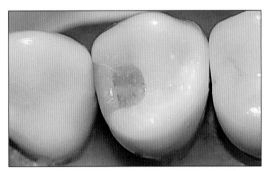
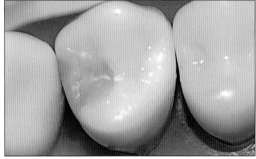

图4-15a　　　　　　　　　　　　　　　图4-15b

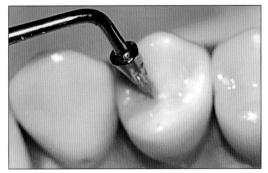
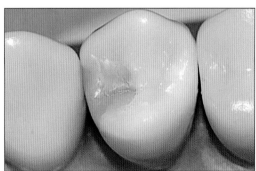

图4-15c　　　　　　　　　　　　　　　图4-15d

7. 使用盘–爪状雕刻刀雕刻殆面剩余部分（图4–16）。三角嵴的斜度对最终结果有着巨大的影响。模仿殆面未预备部分的三角嵴。模仿殆面未预备部分来雕刻副沟。

7. Proceed to carve the rest of the occlusal surface using the discoid-cleoid carver (Fig 4-16). The slope of the triangular ridges have a huge effect on the final outcome.Mimic the triangular ridges on the unprepared part of the occlusal surface. Carve supplemental grooves similar to the unprepared side of the occlusal surface.

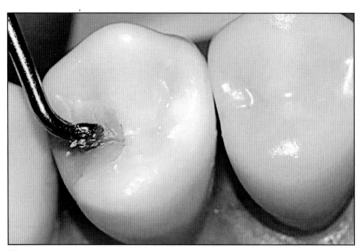

图4-16

8. 雕刻近中沟，它是中央沟的延续，跨过近中边缘嵴，在近中面短距离终止（图4–17a）。然后使用尼龙布抛光最终蜡型（图4–17b和c）。

8. Carve the mesial marginal developmental groove, which is a continuation of the central groove, crossing the mesial marginal ridge and terminating shortly on the mesial surface (Fig 4-17a). Then polish the final wax-up with a nylon stocking (Figs 4-17b and 4-17c).

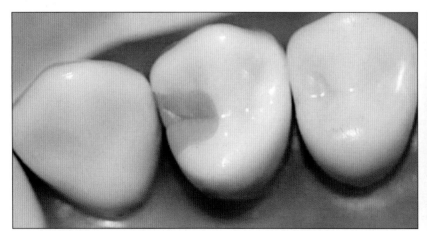

图4-17a　最终蜡型殆面观
Occlusal view of final wax-up.

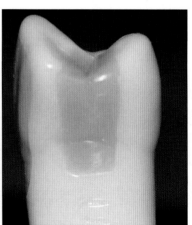

图4-17b　最终蜡型邻面观
Proximal view of final wax-up.

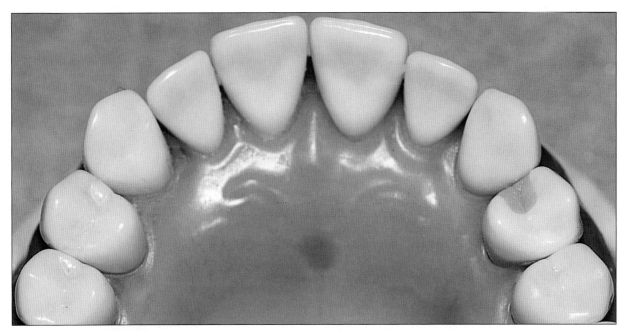

图4-17c　最终蜡型殆面观
Occlusal view of final wax-up.

#24全冠蜡型堆塑步骤

前磨牙全冠蜡型堆塑比前牙蜡型堆塑需要更多的技巧（图4-18）。学习前磨牙殆面堆塑和雕刻是为更复杂的磨牙殆面解剖堆塑打基础。取出#24开始滴蜡堆塑。这一步仍需在牙列模型内外操作。需要两个牙列模型来帮助调整牙尖高度。

Waxing Steps for Tooth #24 Full-Crown Wax-Up

Waxing full premolars requires more skill than waxing anterior teeth (Fig 4-18). Learning how to wax and carve the occlusal surface of premolars should prepare you for waxing the more complex occlusal anatomy of molars. Unscrew tooth #24 to start your wax-up. We are still working in and out of the dentoform. You will need both dentoform arches to aid in adjusting the cusp height.

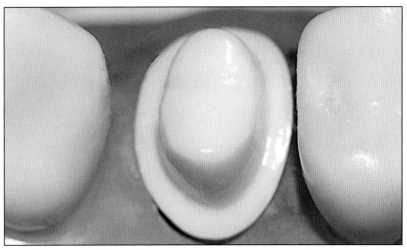

图4-18

1. 形成初始蜡层。

- 手握可摘代模，开始在可摘代模的牙体预备区加蜡。因为前磨牙比前牙大，所以要涂一层较厚的初始蜡层。蜡层厚度均匀，不留空隙（图4-19a和b）
- 延长蜡层超过终止线，以确保蜡层边缘没有缺陷（图4-19c）
- 使用Hollenback雕刻刀雕刻蜡型，使之与终止线平齐且轮廓合适，以实现与可摘代模的平滑过渡（图4-19d）

1. Establish the initial layer of wax.

- With the tooth peg in your hand, start adding wax to cover the prepared area of the tooth peg. A thicker initial layer of wax is applied given that premolars are larger than anterior teeth. The wax should have even thickness with no voids (Figs 4-19a and 4-19b).
- Extend the wax past the finish line. This is done to ensure that the wax is not deficient at the margin (Fig 4-19c).
- Use the Hollenback carver to carve the wax flush with the finish line and with the proper contour to achieve a smooth transition with the tooth peg (Fig 4-19d).

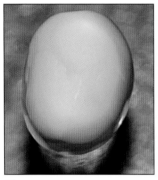 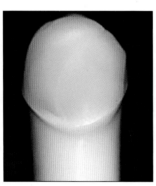 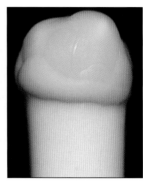 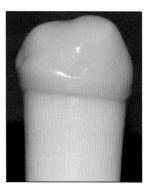

图4-19a　　　　　　图4-19b　　　　　　图4-19c　　　　　　图4-19d

2. 形成邻接关系。

- 将可摘代模放回牙列模型中，并在邻牙上标记近中接触区的位置（图4-20a）。远中接触区位于#23的中1/3处，近中接触区位于#25的殆1/3和中1/3交界处。两个邻面接触区都位于唇舌径/颊舌径中央偏唇/颊侧
- 添加蜡锥，将蜡型和邻牙上的标记连接起来。继续加蜡，直到蜡锥与标记牢固接触（图4-20b和c）

2. Establish proximal contacts.

- Return the tooth to the dentoform and mark the location for the proximal contacts on the adjacent teeth (Fig 4-20a). Distal contact on tooth #23 is at the middle third, and mesial contact on tooth #25 is at the junction of the occlusal and middle thirds. Both contacts are facial to the center of the crown faciolingually.
- Add wax cones to connect your wax-up with the marks on the adjacent teeth. Continue adding wax until the cones make firm contact with the marks (Figs 4-20b and 4-20c).

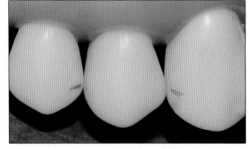 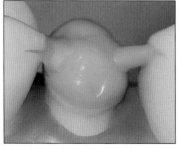 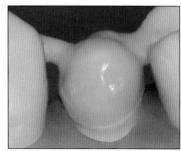

图4-20a　　　　　　图4-20b　唇面观
　　　　　　　　　　　　　　　Labial view.

图4-20c　舌面观
Lingual view.

3. 形成邻面接触区。

- 后牙邻面的颊舌径比前牙邻面的唇舌径更大。因此，在加蜡过程中会产生更宽的邻面。将可摘代模从牙列模型中取出，继续在邻面接触区加蜡至龈方终止线，保持蜡表面相对平坦（图4-21a和b）。然后将蜡延伸至覆盖整个邻面（图4-21c）

- 在颊面和舌面涂一层蜡，使可摘代模周围的蜡厚度均匀（图4-21d）

- 使用Hollenback雕刻刀清除多余的蜡，并从龈方和颊舌面往接触区方向将邻面雕刻平坦。应注意避免雕刻接触区

- 将可摘代模放回牙列模型中，并在殆龈向、颊舌向上检查接触区的位置和密合情况（图4-21e和f）。使用Hollenback雕刻刀清除填塞在颊楔状隙或舌楔状隙的多余的蜡

3. Wax the proximal surface.

- The proximal surfaces of posterior teeth have a larger buccolingual dimension than those of anterior teeth. Therefore, a wider proximal surface is created during waxing. Remove the tooth from the dentoform, and add wax to join the waxed proximal contact to the gingival finish line, keeping the wax relatively flat (Figs 4-21a and 4-21b). Then extend the wax to cover the entire proximal surface (Fig 4-21c).

- Apply a layer of wax to the buccal and lingual surfaces to make the thickness of the wax even around the tooth peg (Fig 4-21d).

- Use your Hollenback carver to remove excess wax and carve the proximal surfaces flat cervical to the contact and buccolingually. Care should be taken to avoid carving the contact.

- Return the tooth to the dentoform and verify the location and closure of the proximal contacts in the occlusogingival and buccolingual directions (Figs 4-21e and 4-21f). Excess wax blocking the buccal or lingual embrasures may be carved at this step with the Hollenback carver.

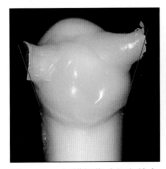

图4-21a　加蜡部位（红色线）

Red lines show where wax is added.

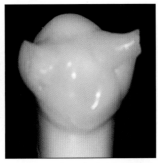

图4-21b　与龈方终止线相连接

Connect contact with gingival finish line.

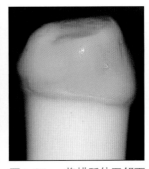

图4-21c　将蜡延伸至邻面

Extend the wax over the proximal surface.

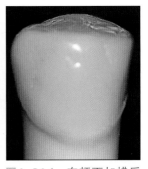

图4-21d　在颊面加蜡后的形态

After adding wax to the buccal surface.

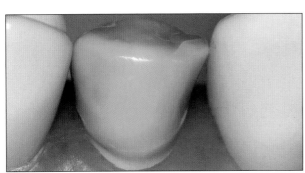

图4-21e

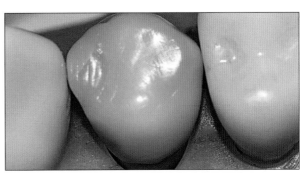

图4-21f

4. 形成殆面边界（牙尖顶、牙尖嵴和边缘嵴）。

- 形成牙尖顶。保持可摘代模在牙列模型中，添加蜡锥将颊尖牙尖顶和舌尖牙尖顶放置在适当的位置，并保持适当的高度。**位置**：颊尖牙尖顶与第二前磨牙颊尖牙尖顶处于同一水平或略偏颊侧，舌尖牙尖顶比第二前磨牙舌尖牙尖顶更偏舌侧（图4-22a）。正确放置颊尖和舌尖牙尖顶对于形成正确尺寸的殆面非常重要。颊尖牙尖顶略偏远中，舌尖牙尖顶略偏近中。在最终的雕刻和修形步骤中，进一步调整牙尖顶位置。**高度**：颊尖比第二前磨牙颊尖略长，比尖牙牙尖略短（图4-22b）。舌尖几乎与上颌第二前磨牙的舌尖等高。模仿对侧同名牙的牙尖高度。当蜡型仍然温热时，将上颌牙列和下颌牙列合在一起可以帮助调整舌尖的高度（图4-22c）。如果蜡锥很高，它会在碰到对颌边缘嵴时变平。然后可以通过雕刻来平整表面

4. Establish the boundaries of the occlusal surface (cusp tips, cusp rides, and marginal ridges).

- Form the cusp tips. With the tooth in the dentoform, add wax cones to place the buccal and lingual cusp tips at their proper location and with the approximate proper height. **Location:** The buccal cusp tip is in the same level or slightly buccal to the buccal cusp tip of the second premolar, and the lingual cusp tip is lingual to the lingual cusp of the second premolar (Fig 4-22a). Properly placing the buccal and lingual cusp tips is very important to create an occlusal surface with the right dimensions. The buccal cusp tip is positioned slightly distally, and the lingual cusp tip is positioned slightly mesially. Further adjustment of the cusp tip location is done in the final carving and contouring step. **Height:** The buccal cusp is slightly longer than the buccal cusp of the second premolar and slightly shorter than the canine cusp (Fig 4-22b). The lingual cusp is almost the same height as the lingual cusp of the maxillary second premolar. Mimic the cusp height of the contralateral first premolar. Closing the maxillary and mandibular arches together when the wax is still warm can help you adjust the height of the lingual cusp (Fig 4-22c). If your wax cone is high, it will become flattened on touching the opposing marginal ridge. Then the flat surface can be adjusted by carving.

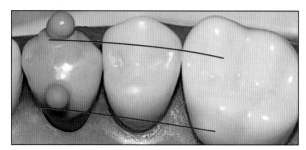

图4-22a 牙尖顶平面（红色线）
Plane of cusp tips *(red lines)*.

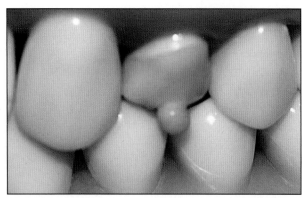

图4-22b

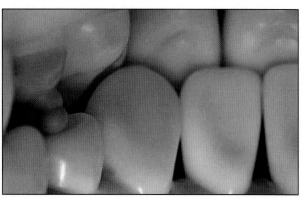

图4-22c

- 形成牙尖嵴。牙尖嵴从牙尖顶向近中和远中倾斜，形成𬌗面的颊舌边界。加蜡将蜡型的近中边界连接到相应的牙尖顶，形成牙尖嵴，而不影响牙尖高度（图4-22d）。每次加蜡都要从近中边界向牙尖顶拖动蜡滴。舌尖比颊尖更圆钝（图4-22e和f）。给颊尖牙尖嵴加蜡时，多余的蜡可能会接触到邻牙，可以使用Hollenback雕刻刀清除。考虑到牙齿的舌向聚合，舌尖牙尖嵴的蜡不会接触到邻牙

- 形成边缘嵴。加蜡将颊尖的近端连接到相应的舌尖牙尖嵴。这将形成𬌗面的六边形轮廓。颊尖牙尖顶略偏远中，舌尖牙尖顶略偏近中（图4-22g）。通常，相邻的边缘嵴必须具有相同的高度

- Establish the cusp ridges. Cusp ridges slope from the cusp tips mesially and distally, forming the buccal and lingual boundaries of the occlusal surface. Apply wax to connect the proximal boundaries of your wax-up to the corresponding cusp tip to form the cusp ridges, without interfering with the cusp heights achieved (Fig 4-22d). Each wax increment is dragged starting at the proximal boundary and ending at the cusp tip. The lingual cusp ridges are more rounded than the buccal cusp ridges (Figs 4-22e and 4-22f). When waxing the buccal cusp ridges, excess wax may contact the adjacent teeth, which can be removed with the Hollenback carver. The lingual cusp ridge wax does not contact the adjacent teeth given the lingual convergence of the teeth.

- Establish the marginal ridges. Apply wax to connect the proximal ends of the buccal cusp ridges to the corresponding lingual cusp ridges. This will create the hexagonal outline of the occlusal surface. The buccal cusp tip is slightly distal and the lingual cusp tip is slightly mesial(Fig 4-22g). As a rule, the adjacent marginal ridges *must* be the same height.

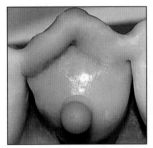 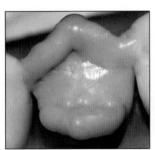 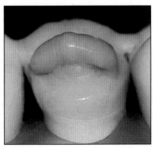 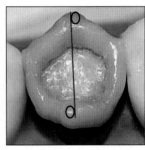

图4-22d　　　　图4-22e　　　　图4-22f　　　　图4-22g

5. 堆塑颊面。

- 在颊面加蜡，完成颊面轮廓。在颈1/3处添加更多的蜡，形成外形高点。然后通过将颊面外形高点的近中边界和远中边界与相应的牙尖嵴相连而形成线角。通过将颊面外形高点𬌗方部分连接到牙尖顶而形成颊轴嵴（图4-23a）。这些隆起在上颌第一前磨牙上非常明显。保持可摘代模在牙列模型中，添加颊面轮廓，以实现精确定位

5. Wax the buccal surface.

- Add wax to the buccal surface to complete the buccal contour. More wax is applied at the cervical third to form the height of contour. The line angles are then waxed by joining the mesial and distal ends of the buccal height of contour to the corresponding cusp ridges. The buccal ridge is created by connecting the occlusal part of the buccal height of contour to the cusp tip (Fig 4-23a). These elevations are quite prominent on the maxillary first premolar. The contours are added with the tooth in the dentoform for precise localization.

- 使用堆蜡工具在剩余区域加蜡（图4-23b）。这可以通过将可摘代模放回牙列模型中或从牙列模型中取出可摘代模来完成
- 清除多余的蜡以获得光滑的颊面，使线角、外形高点、颊轴嵴保持位置和轮廓适当（图4-23c）。使用盘-爪状雕刻刀雕刻发育沟，与对侧同名牙上的发育沟保持一致。从𬌗面观来看，线角和颊轴嵴的位置和轮廓应与对侧同名牙一致

- Fill in the remaining areas with wax using your wax-addition instruments (Fig 4-23b). This can be done with the tooth inside or outside the dentoform.
- Carve the excess wax to achieve a smooth buccal surface, maintaining the proper position and contour of the line angles, height of contour, and buccal ridge (Fig 4-23c). The developmental depressions may be carved with the discoid-cleoid carver to match the depressions on the contralateral first premolar. Line angles and the buccal ridge should conform in position and contour to those on the contralateral first premolar, when viewed from the occlusal view.

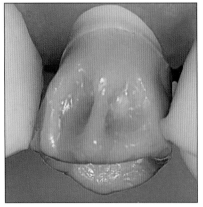

图4-23a 添加轮廓线

Add contours.

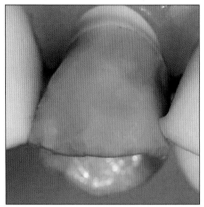

图4-23b 充填剩余区域

Fill the remaining areas.

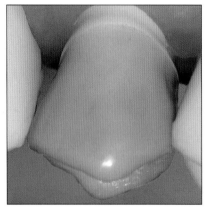

图4-23c 修形和平整

Carve and smooth.

6. 堆塑舌面。

- 舌面加一层蜡，完成舌面轮廓。在中1/3处添加更多的蜡，形成外形高点。然后通过将舌面外形高点的近中边界和远中边界与相应的牙尖嵴相连而形成线角。通过将舌面外形高点𬌗方部分与牙尖顶相连而形成舌轴嵴（图4-24a）。舌侧线角不如颊侧线角明显，整个舌面相当突出。保持可摘代模在牙列模型中，添加舌面轮廓，以实现精确定位。线角和舌轴嵴的位置和轮廓应与对侧同名牙一致
- 使用堆蜡工具在剩余区域加蜡（图4-24b）。这可以通过将可摘代模放回牙列模型中或从牙列模型中取出可摘代模来完成
- 清除多余的蜡以获得光滑的舌面，使线角、外形高点、舌轴嵴保持位置和轮廓适当（图4-24c）

6. Wax the lingual surface.

- Add wax to the lingual surface to complete the lingual contour. More wax is applied at the middle third to form the height of contour. The line angles are then waxed by joining the mesial and distal ends of the lingual height of contour to the corresponding cusp ridges. The lingual ridge is created by connecting the occlusal part of the lingual height of contour to the cusp tip (Fig 4-24a). The lingual line angles are less prominent than the buccal line angles, and the entire lingual surface is quite convex. The contours are added with the tooth in the dentoform for precise localization. Line angles and lingual ridge should conform in position and contour to those of the contralateral first premolar.
- Fill in the remaining areas with wax using your wax-addition instruments (Fig 4-24b). This can be done with the tooth outside of the dentoform.
- Carve the excess wax to achieve a smooth lingual surface, maintaining the proper position and countour of the line angles, height of contour, and lingual ridge (Fig 4-24c).

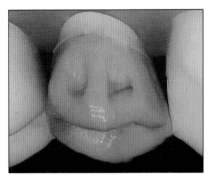

图4-24a　添加轮廓线

Add contours.

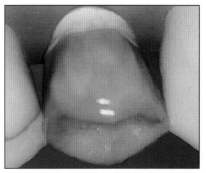

图4-24b　充填剩余区域

Fill the remaining areas.

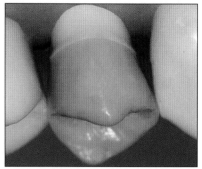

图4-24c　修形和平整

Carve and smooth.

7. 形成三角嵴，完成殆面。

- 加蜡将牙尖顶连接到殆面的中心，形成颊尖和舌尖的三角嵴（图4-25a和b）。从邻面观可以最直观地观察到，上颌第一前磨牙呈现出非常陡峭的三角嵴

- 在三角嵴的近中面和远中面添加更多的蜡，以完成殆面（图4-25c和d）

7. Establish the triangular ridges and complete the occlusal surface.

- Apply wax to connect the cusp tips to the center of the occlusal surface, forming the triangular ridges of the buccal and lingual cusps (Figs 4-25a and 4-25b). The maxillary first premolar exhibits triangular ridges that are quite steep. This is best visualized from a proximal view.

- Add more wax mesial and distal to the ridges you created to complete the occlusal surface (Figs 4-25c and 4-25d).

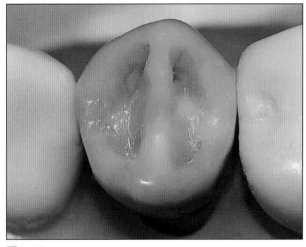

图4-25a

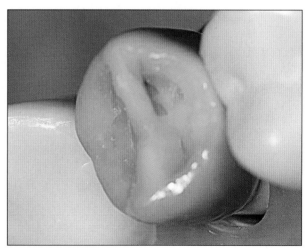

图4-25b

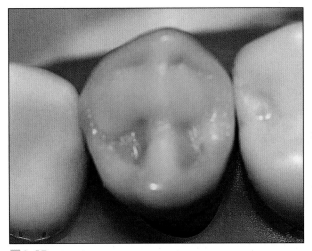

图4-25c

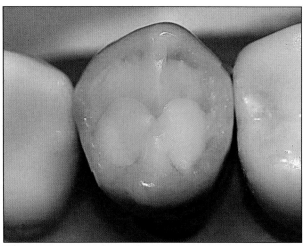

图4-25d

8. 雕刻𬌗面。

• 首先使用橡子形抛光器标记中央沟的位置，中央沟应与上颌第二前磨牙中央沟成一直线（图4-26a）

• 使用盘–爪状雕刻刀的小工作尖雕刻锥形的牙尖。每个牙尖从牙尖顶向中央沟延伸，从三角嵴向近中边界和远中边界倾斜（形似金字塔；图4-26b）

• 按照与相邻边缘嵴相同的高度雕刻边缘嵴。使用Hollenback雕刻刀、盘–爪状雕刻刀来调整边缘嵴的宽度和轮廓。使用尼龙布磨圆、抛光边缘嵴

• 雕刻与对侧同名牙一致的中央沟，需要在继续雕刻𬌗面时对其进行几次改进

• 使用橡子形抛光器或Hollenback雕刻刀的工作尖雕刻三角窝。如果边缘嵴和牙尖堆塑适当，只需要微调即可形成三角窝

• 使用橡子形抛光器雕刻近中沟，并将其延伸至近中面一小段距离

• 雕刻与对侧同名牙一致的副沟

• 根据需要精修颊楔状隙、舌楔状隙，使其大小和位置与对侧同名牙一致

• 使用注射器吹气或刷子清除𬌗面上多余的蜡屑

• 使用尼龙布抛光𬌗面。棉签可以和长袜一起用来抛光𬌗面窝沟

8. Carve the occlusal surface.

• Start by marking the location of the central groove with the acorn burnisher. The central groove should be in line with the central groove of the maxillary second premolar (Fig 4-26a).

• Use the small discoid-cleoid carver to carve the pyramidal shape of the cusps. Each cusp slopes from the cusp tip to the central groove and from the triangular ridges toward the mesial and distal sides (like a pyramid; Fig 4-26b).

• Carve the marginal ridges at the same level as the adjacent marginal ridges. Adjust their width and contour with the Hollenback and discoid-cleoid carvers. A nylon stocking is used to contour and polish the ridges.

• Carve the central groove identical to that on the contralateral first premolar, you may need to refine it a few times as you continue to carve the occlusal surface.

• Carve the triangular fossae with the acorn burnisher or the tip of the Hollenback carver. If you achieve properly contoured marginal ridges and cusps, the triangular fossae can be easily emphasized with minimal carving.

• Carve the mesial marginal groove with the acorn burnisher, and extend it onto the mesial surface for a short distance.

• Carve supplemental grooves identical to those on the contralateral first premolar.

• Refine the buccal and lingual embrasures as needed, so that they are consistent in size and location with those on the contralateral premolar.

• Remove wax flakes on the occlusal surface using an airway syringe or a brush.

• Polish the occlusal surface with a nylon stocking. A cotton swab can be used with a stocking to polish the depressions on the surface.

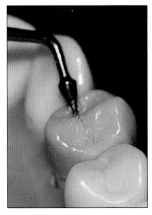

图4-26a

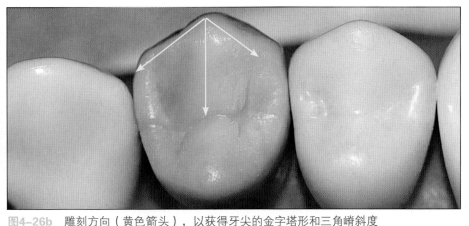

图4-26b　雕刻方向（黄色箭头），以获得牙尖的金字塔形和三角嵴斜度

The direction of carving *(yellow arrows)* to achieve the pyramidal shape of the cusps and the slope of the triangular ridges.

9. 完成最终的雕刻和修形。

- 从不同角度检查线角、点角、楔状隙、邻面接触区、牙尖嵴、殆面解剖结构、外形高点和终止线。根据需要进行加蜡和雕刻，来最终实现蜡型形态与对侧同名牙一致（图4-27a~d）

- 将可摘代模从牙列模型中取出，并与未预备的可摘代模比对。从邻面观来观察牙齿，确保颊面外形高点位于颈1/3处，舌面外形高点位于中1/3处。确保三角嵴的斜度以及蜡型与终止线平滑过渡（图4-27e和f）

9. Complete final carving and contouring.

- Line angles, point angles, embrasures, proximal contacts, cusp ridges, occlusal anatomy, heights of contour, and finish line are all checked from different views. Wax addition and carving is done as needed to achieve a wax-up that is consistent with the contralateral premolar (Figs 4-27a to 4-27d).

- Remove the tooth from the dentoform and compare it to the unprepared dentoform tooth. View the tooth from a proximal view to verify that the buccal height of contour is at the cervical third and the lingual height of contour is at the middle third. Verify the steep slope of the triangular ridges and that the wax is in smooth transition with the finish line (Figs 4-27e and 4-27f).

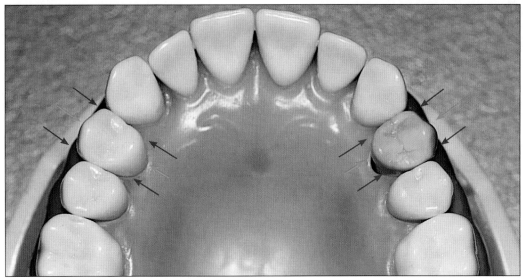

图4-27a　最好从殆面观来观察颊侧线角、舌侧线角（红色箭头）以及颊轴嵴、舌轴嵴（绿色箭头），位置和轮廓应与对侧同名牙一致。颊侧线角和颊轴嵴比舌侧更明显

Buccal and lingual line angles *(red arrows)* and buccal and lingual ridges *(green arrows)* are best visualized from the occlusal view and should conform in position and contour to those of the contralateral premolar. The buccal line angles and buccal ridge are more prominent than their lingual counterparts.

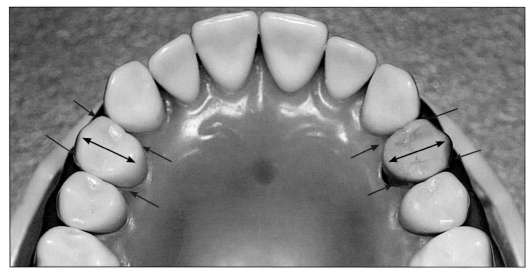

图4-27b　最好从𬌗面观来观察点角（红色箭头），位置和轮廓应与对侧同名牙一致。从𬌗面观来观察时，蜡型的颊舌径（黑色箭头）应该与对侧同名牙一致

Point angles *(red arrows)* are best visualized from the occlusal view and should conform in position and contour to the contralateral tooth. The buccolingual dimension of the tooth *(black arrows)* should be identical to the contralateral premolar when viewed occlusally.

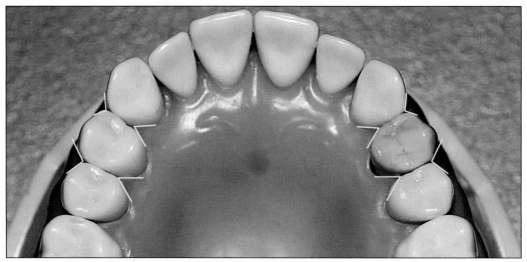

图4-27c　从𬌗面观来观察颊楔状隙和舌楔状隙（黄色标记），大小、位置应与对侧楔状隙一致

The buccal and lingual embrasures *(in yellow)* are visualized from the occlusal view and should match the contralateral embrasures in size and location.

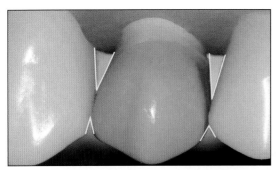

图4-27d 从颊面观或舌面观来观察𬌗楔状隙和颈邻间隙（黄色标记），大小、位置应与对侧楔状隙一致

Occlusal and cervical embrasures *(in yellow)* are visualized from a buccal or lingual view and should match the contralateral embrasures in size and location.

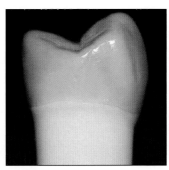

图4-27e 远中邻面观

Distal view.

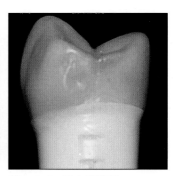

图4-27f 近中邻面观

Mesial view.

10. 完成最终的平整和抛光。

- 使用雕刻刀修平表面，使用尼龙布轻轻抛光。这会使蜡型表面高度抛光（图4-28）。应避免长时间抛光，因为这样可能会改变牙齿的解剖结构。为了避免破坏蜡型，请勿过度加压。使用注射器吹气或刷子清除蜡型和牙列模型上的蜡屑

10. Complete final smoothing and polishing.

- Plane the surface with a carver, and buff lightly with a nylon stocking. This should give your wax-up a nice polished appearance (Fig 4-28). Avoid lengthy polishing because it may change the tooth anatomy. Use only gentle pressure to avoid breaking your wax-up. Remove wax flakes on your wax-up and dentoform using an airway syringe or a brush.

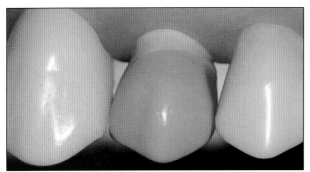

图4-28a 最终蜡型颊面观

Buccal view of final wax-up.

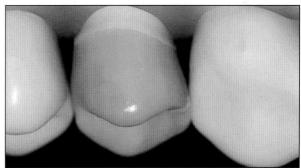

图4-28b 最终蜡型舌面观

Lingual view of final wax-up.

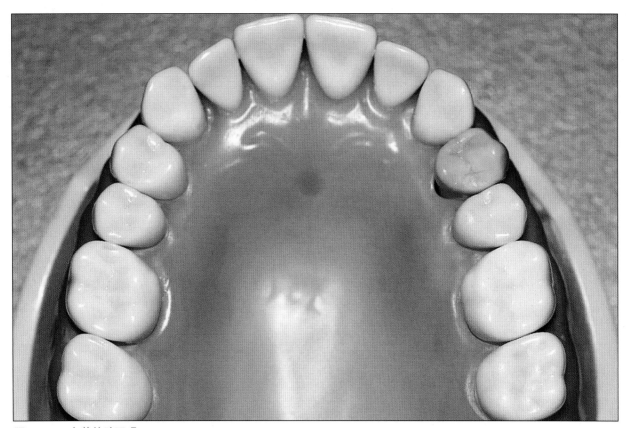

图4-28c 完整的殆面观
Complete occlusal view.

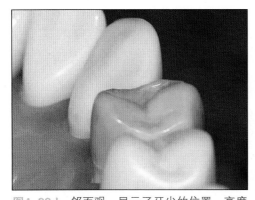

图4-28d 邻面观，显示了牙尖的位置、高度
和三角嵴斜度

Proximal view showing cusp alignment,
height, and slope of triangular ridges.

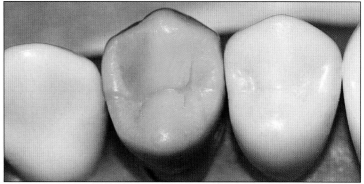

图4-28e

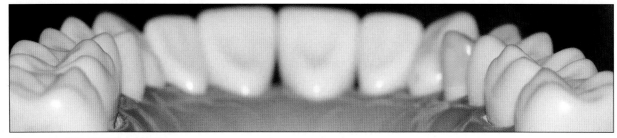

图4-28f 最终蜡型远中邻面观
Distal view of final wax-up.

下颌第二前磨牙全冠蜡型堆塑的形态和标准[6-7]

Morphology and Criteria for Mandibular Second Premolar Full-Crown Wax-Up[6,7]

颊面观

从颊面观可以观察到（图4-29a）：

- 外形呈梯形
- 从颊面观来看，牙冠显得又短又大
- 颊面光滑凸起
- 颊尖比下颌第一前磨牙颊尖短
- 颊尖牙尖顶钝，偏近中
- 颊尖的近中牙尖嵴比远中牙尖嵴短
- 颊轴嵴是从颊面外形高点延伸至牙尖顶的隆起
- 颊轴嵴的近中和远中有两条浅的纵向发育沟
- 近中和远中接触区位于殆1/3处
- 殆楔状隙和颈邻间隙与对侧同名牙一致

舌面观

从舌面观可以观察到（图4-29b）：

- 舌尖比颊尖短，但比下颌第一前磨牙的舌尖长
- 舌面在近远中向和殆颈向均有凸起
- 观察到的舌向聚合程度比下颌第一前磨牙更小
- 近中舌尖几乎占近远中径的2/3
- 远中舌尖比近中舌尖短，并通过一条明显的舌沟与近中舌尖分开，舌沟延伸至舌面一小段距离
- 殆楔状隙和颈邻间隙与对侧同名牙一致

Buccal view

The following can be observed in the buccal view (Fig 4-29a):

- Trapezoidal outline.
- Crown appears short and bulky from buccal aspect.
- Buccal surface smooth and convex.
- Buccal cusp shorter than that of the mandibular first premolar.
- Buccal cusp tip is blunt and positioned mesially.
- Mesial cusp ridge of the buccal cusp shorter than the distal cusp ridge.
- Buccal ridge is a prominent elevation and extends from the buccal height of contour to the cusp tip.
- Two shallow longitudinal depressions exist mesial and distal to the buccal ridge.
- Mesial and distal proximal contacts located at the occlusal third.
- Occlusal and cervical embrasures consistent with those of the contralateral premolar.

Lingual view

The following can be observed in the lingual view (Fig 4-29b):

- Lingual cusps shorter than the buccal cusp but longer than the lingual cusp of the mandibular first premolar.
- Lingual surface convex mesiodistally and occlusocervically.
- Less lingual convergence than that observed in the mandibular first premolar.
- Mesiolingual cusp nearly two-thirds the mesiodistal width.
- Distolingual cusp shorter than and separated from the mesiolingual cusp by a distinct lingual groove, which runs a very short distance on the lingual surface.
- Occlusal and cervical embrasures consistent with those of the contralateral premolar.

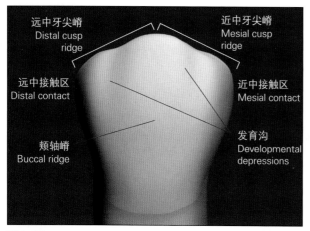

图4-29a

远中牙尖嵴
Distal cusp
ridge

近中牙尖嵴
Mesial cusp
ridge

远中接触区
Distal contact

近中接触区
Mesial contact

颊轴嵴
Buccal ridge

发育沟
Developmental
depressions

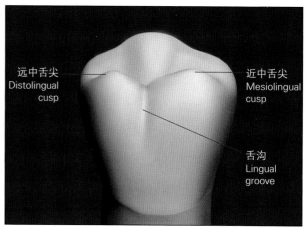

图4-29b

远中舌尖
Distolingual
cusp

近中舌尖
Mesiolingual
cusp

舌沟
Lingual
groove

邻面观

从邻面观可以观察到（图4-29c和d）：

- 外形呈菱形
- 牙冠相对于牙根向舌侧倾斜
- 颊尖牙尖顶钝，且颊尖比舌尖长
- 颊面外形高点位于颈1/3处，舌面外形高点位于中1/3处
- 三角嵴显著，从牙尖顶延伸至中央沟
- 颊舌径与对侧同名牙一致

殆面观

从殆面观可以观察到（图4-29e）：

- 外形呈方形
- 颊舌径比近远中径略大
- 殆面形态由一个突出的颊尖、两个舌尖（通常）、牙尖嵴、三角嵴、边缘嵴、窝（中央窝和两个三角窝）和沟组成
- 发育沟汇聚在中央窝，形成Y字形
- 边缘嵴与相邻边缘嵴处于同一水平
- 舌向聚合程度比下颌第一前磨牙更小

Proximal view

The following can be observed in the proximal views (Figs 4-29c and 4-29d):

- Rhomboidal outline.
- Crown lingually inclined in relation to the root.
- Buccal cusp tip blunt and the buccal cusp longer than the lingual cusps.
- Buccal height of contour located at the cervical third, and lingual height of contour located at the middle third.
- Triangular ridges well developed and convex from the cusp tip to the central groove.
- Buccolingual dimension of the tooth consistent with that of the contralateral premolar.

Occlusal view

The following can be observed in the occlusal view (Fig 4-29e):

- Square outline.
- Buccolingual dimension of the crown slightly greater than the mesiodistal dimension.
- Occlusal morphology includes a prominent buccal cusp, two lingual cusps (usually), cusp ridges, triangular ridges, marginal ridges, occlusal fossae (central fossa and two triangular fossae), and grooves.
- Developmental grooves converge in the central pit forming a Y-shape.
- Marginal ridges at the same level as the adjacent marginal ridges.
- Exhibits less lingual convergence than the mandibular first premolar.

- 线角及点角的位置和轮廓与对侧同名牙一致
- 舌侧线角不如颊侧线角明显
- 颊楔状隙、舌楔状隙的大小和位置与对侧同名牙一致

- Line angles and point angles consistent in position and contour to those of the contralateral premolar.
- Lingual line angles less prominent than the buccal line angles.
- Buccal and lingual embrasures consistent in size and location with those of the contralateral premolar.

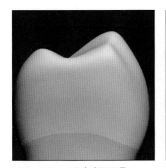

图4-29c 近中邻面观 Mesial view.

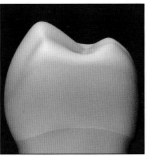

图4-29d 远中邻面观 Distal view.

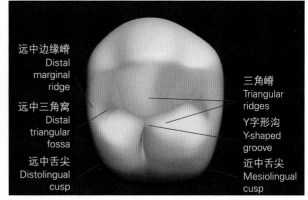

远中边缘嵴 Distal marginal ridge

远中三角窝 Distal triangular fossa

远中舌尖 Distolingual cusp

三角嵴 Triangular ridges

Y字形沟 Y-shaped groove

近中舌尖 Mesiolingual cusp

图4-29e

#35全冠蜡型堆塑步骤

注意对侧同名牙，即#45解剖形态。取出#35开始滴蜡堆塑。这一步仍需在牙列模型内外操作（图4-30）。需要两个牙列模型来帮助调整牙尖高度。

Waxing Steps for Tooth #35 Full-Crown Wax-Up

Notice the anatomy of your contralateral tooth #45. Unscrew tooth #35 to start your waxing. We are still working in and out of the dentoform, but most of the steps are done with the tooth inside the dentoform (Fig 4-30). You may use both arches to adjust the cusp height.

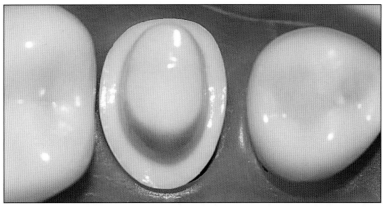

图4-30

1. 形成初始蜡层。

- 手握可摘代模，开始在可摘代模的牙体预备区加蜡。因为前磨牙比前牙大，所以要涂一层较厚的初始蜡层。蜡层厚度均匀，不留空隙（图4-31a）

- 延长蜡层超过终止线（图4-31b），以确保蜡层边缘没有缺陷

- 使用Hollenback雕刻刀雕刻蜡型，使之与终止线平齐且轮廓合适，以实现与可摘代模的平滑过渡（图4-31c）

1. Establish the initial layer of wax.

- With the tooth peg in your hand, start adding wax to cover the prepared area of the tooth peg. A thicker initial layer of wax is applied because premolars are larger than anterior teeth. The wax should be even in thickness and have no voids (Fig 4-31a).

- Extend the wax past the finish line (Fig 4-31b) to ensure that the wax is not deficient at the margin.

- Use the Hollenback carver to carve the wax flush with the finish line and with the proper contour to achieve a smooth transition with the tooth peg (Fig 4-31c).

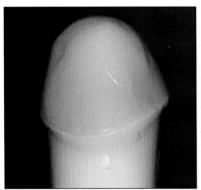

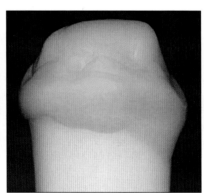
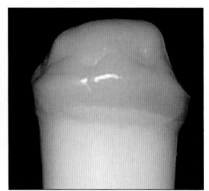

图4-31a   图4-31b   图4-31c

2. 形成邻接关系。

- 将可摘代模放回牙列模型中，并在邻牙上标记近中接触区的位置（图4-32a）。两个接触区都在𬌗1/3处

- 添加蜡锥，将蜡型和邻牙上的标记连接起来（图4-32b和c）

2. Establish the proximal contacts.

- Mark the location for the proximal contacts on the adjacent teeth and return the wax-up to the dentoform (Fig 4-32a). Both contacts are at the occlusal thirds.

- Add wax cones to connect your wax-up with the marks on the adjacent teeth (Figs 4-32b and 4-32c).

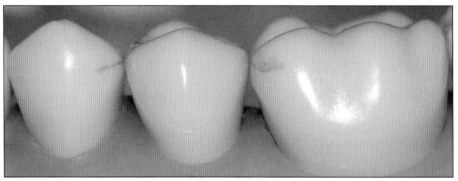

图4-32a

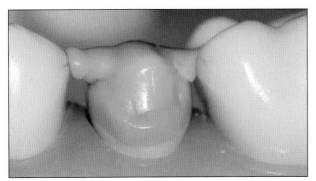

图4-32b 颊面观
Buccal view.

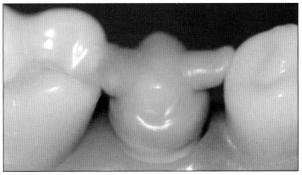

图4-32c 舌面观
Lingual view.

3. 形成邻面接触区。

- 后牙的邻面比前牙的邻面有更大的颊舌径，因此上蜡时会产生更宽的邻面。将可摘代模从牙列模型中取出，继续在邻面接触区加蜡至龈方终止线，保持蜡表面相对平坦，然后将蜡延伸至覆盖整个邻面（图4-33a和b）

- 在颊面和舌面涂一层蜡，使可摘代模周围的蜡厚度均匀（图4-33c和d）

- 使用Hollenback雕刻刀清除多余的蜡，并从𬌗龈方和颊舌面往接触区方向将邻面雕刻平坦。所有邻面舌向聚合，但下颌第二前磨牙比下颌第一前磨牙舌向聚合程度小

- 将可摘代模放回牙列模型中，并在𬌗龈向、颊舌向上检查接触区的位置和密合情况（图4-33e~g）

- 使用Hollenback雕刻刀清除填塞在颊楔状隙或舌楔状隙的多余的蜡（图4-33h和i）

3. Wax the proximal surface.

- The proximal surfaces of posterior teeth have a larger buccolingual dimension than those of anterior teeth, therefore a wider proximal surface is created during waxing. Remove the tooth from the dentoform, add wax to join the waxed proximal contact to the gingival finish line while keeping the wax relatively flat, and then extend the wax to cover the entire proximal surface (Figs 4-33a and 4-33b).

- Apply a layer of wax to the buccal and lingual surfaces to make the thickness of the wax even around the tooth peg (Figs 4-33c and 4-33d).

- Use your Hollenback carver to remove excess wax and carve the proximal surfaces flat cervical to the contact and buccolingually. All proximal surfaces converge lingually but the mandibular second premolar exhibits less lingual convergence than the mandibular first premolar.

- Return the tooth to the dentoform and verify the location and closure of the proximal contacts in the occlusogingival and buccolingual directions (Figs 4-33e to 4-33g).

- Excess wax blocking the buccal or lingual embrasures may be carved at this step with the Hollenback carver (Figs 4-33h and 4-33i).

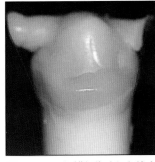

图4-33a 加蜡部位（红色线）
Red lines show where wax is added.

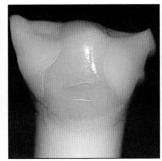

图4-33b 邻面成形后
After forming the proximal surface.

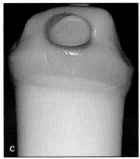

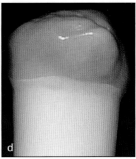

图4-33c和d 邻面观显示加蜡将近中接触区连接到龈方终止线，随后将蜡添加到颊面和舌面
Proximal view showing wax addition to join proximal contact to the gingival finish line and subsequent wax addition to the buccal and lingual surfaces.

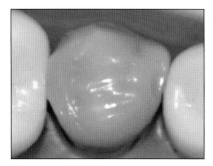
图4-33e 殆面观
Occlusal view.

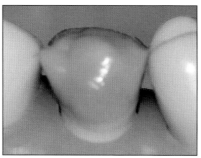
图4-33f 颊面观
Buccal view.

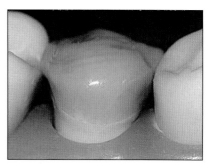
图4-33g 舌面观
Lingual view.

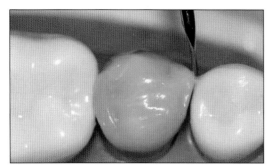
图4-33h

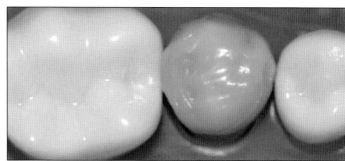
图4-33i

4. 形成殆面边界（牙尖顶、牙尖嵴和边缘嵴）。

- 形成牙尖顶。保持可摘代模在牙列模型中，添加蜡锥将颊尖牙尖顶和舌尖牙尖顶放置在适当的位置，并保持适当的高度（图4-34a）。**位置**：牙尖顶应与邻牙牙尖顶在同一平面。颊尖牙尖顶略偏近中。颊尖最大，近中舌尖比远中舌尖大。**高度**：颊尖比第一前磨牙颊尖略低，外形更圆钝。近中舌尖比颊尖短，但比下颌第一前磨牙的舌尖长且宽。远中舌尖比近中舌尖更短小。当蜡型仍然温热时，将上颌牙列和下颌牙列合在一起可以调整颊尖的高度（图4-34b）。如果牙尖很高，它会在碰到对颌边缘嵴时变平，然后可以通过雕刻来平整表面

4. Wax the boundaries of the occlusal surface (cusp tips, cusp ridges, and marginal ridges).

- Form the cusp tips. With the tooth in the dentoform, add wax cones to place the buccal and lingual cusp tips at their proper location and with the approximate proper height (Fig 4-34a). **Location:** The cusp tips should be in the same plane as those of the adjacent teeth. The buccal cusp tip is positioned slightly mesially. The buccal cusp is the largest and the mesiolingual cusp is larger than the distolingual cusp. **Height:** The buccal cusp is slightly shorter than the buccal cusp of the first premolar and more blunt. The mesiolingual cusp is shorter than the buccal cusp but longer and wider than the lingual cusp of the mandibular first premolar. The distolingual cusp is shorter and smaller than the mesiolingual cusp. Closing the maxillary and mandibular arches together with the wax still warm can help you adjust the height of the buccal cusp (Fig 4-34b). If the cusp is high, it will become flattened on touching the opposing marginal ridge, and then the flat surface can be adjusted by carving.

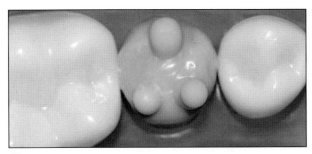

图4-34a

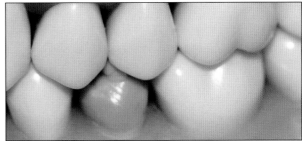

图4-34b

- 形成牙尖嵴。加蜡将蜡型的近中边缘连接到相应的牙尖顶，形成牙尖嵴，而不影响牙尖高度（图4-34c和d）。远中牙尖嵴非常小，只需要添加少量的蜡
- 形成边缘嵴。加蜡将颊尖的近端连接到相应的舌尖牙尖嵴。这将形成𬌗面的六边形轮廓（图4-34e）

- Establish the cusp ridges. Apply wax to connect the proximal boundaries of your wax-up to the corresponding cusp tip to form the cusp ridges, without interfering with the cusp heights achieved (Figs 4-34c and 4-34d). The distolingual cusp ridges are quite small and require only minimal wax addition.
- Establish the marginal ridges. Apply wax to connect the proximal ends of the buccal cusp ridges to the corresponding proximal ends of the lingual cusp ridges to form the marginal ridges. This will create the square outline of the occlusal surface (Fig 4-34e).

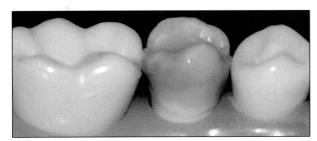

图4-34c

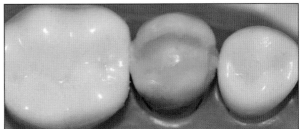

图4-34d

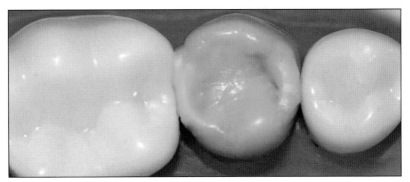

图4-34e

5. 堆塑颊面。

- 在颊面加蜡，完成颊面轮廓。在颈1/3处添加更多的蜡，形成外形高点。然后通过将颊面外形高点的近中边界和远中边界与相应的牙尖嵴相连而形成线角。通过将颊面外形高点牙合方部分连接到牙尖顶形成颊轴嵴。保持可摘代模在牙列模型中，添加颊面轮廓，以实现精确定位（图4-35a）

- 使用堆蜡工具在剩余区域加蜡（图4-35b）。这可以通过将可摘代模放回牙列模型中或从牙列模型中取出可摘代模来完成

- 清除多余的蜡以获得光滑的颊面，使线角、外形高点、颊轴嵴保持位置和轮廓适当（图4-35c）

5. Wax the buccal surface.

- Add wax to the buccal surface to complete the buccal contour. More wax is applied at the cervical third to form the height of contour. The line angles are then waxed by joining the mesial and distal ends of the buccal height of contour to the corresponding cusp ridges. The buccal ridge is created by connecting the occlusal part of the buccal height of contour to the cusp tip. The contours are added with the tooth in the dentoform for precise localization (Fig 4-35a).

- Fill in the remaining areas with wax using your wax-addition instruments (Fig 4-35b). This can be done with the tooth inside or outside of the dentoform.

- Carve the excess wax to achieve a smooth buccal surface, maintaining the proper position and contour of the line angles, height of contour, and buccal ridge (Fig 4-35c).

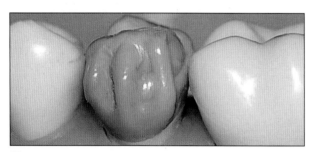

图4-35a

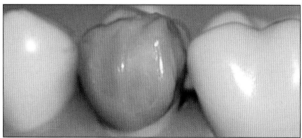

图4-35b

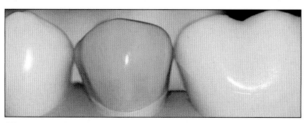

图4-35c

6. 堆塑舌面。

- 舌面加一层蜡，完成舌面轮廓。在中1/3处添加更多的蜡，形成外形高点。然后通过将舌面外形高点的近中边界和远中边界与相应的牙尖嵴相连而形成线角。通过将舌面外形高点牙合方部分与牙尖顶相连而形成舌轴嵴。舌侧线角不如颊侧线角明显，整个舌面相当突出。保持可摘代模在牙列模型中，添加舌面轮廓，以实现

6. Wax the lingual surface.

- Add wax to the lingual surface to complete the lingual contour. More wax is applied at the middle third to form the height of contour. The line angles are then waxed by joining the mesial and distal ends of the lingual height of contour to the corresponding cusp ridges. The lingual ridge is created by connecting the occlusal part of the lingual height of contour to the distal cusp ridge of the mesiolingual cusp. The lingual line angles are less prominent than the buccal line angles, and the entire lingual surface

精确定位。线角、舌轴嵴的位置和轮廓应与对侧同名牙一致（图4-36a）

- 使用堆蜡工具在剩余区域加蜡（图4-36b）。这可以通过将可摘代模放回牙列模型中或从牙列模型中取出可摘代模来完成
- 清除多余的蜡以获得光滑的舌面，使线角、外形高点、舌轴嵴保持位置和轮廓适当（图4-36c）

is quite convex. The contours are added with the tooth in the dentoform for precise localization. Line angles and lingual ridge should conform in position and contour to those on the contralateral second premolar (Fig 4-36a).

- Fill in the remaining areas with wax using your wax-addition instruments (Fig 4-36b). This can be done with the tooth outside of the dentoform.
- Carve the excess wax to achieve a smooth lingual surface, maintaining the proper position and contour of the line angles, height of contour, and lingual ridge (Fig 4-36c).

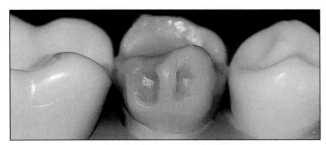

图4-36a

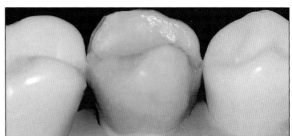

图4-36b

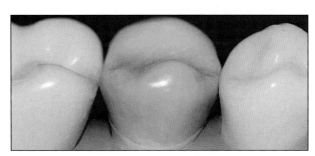

图4-36c

7. 形成三角嵴，完成𬌗面。
- 加蜡将牙尖顶连接到𬌗面的中心，形成颊尖和舌尖的三角嵴（图4-37a）。下颌第二前磨牙有凸起的三角嵴
- 在三角嵴的近中面和远中面添加更多的蜡，以完成𬌗面（图4-37b）

7. Establish the triangular ridges and complete the occlusal surface.
- Apply wax to connect the cusp tips to the center of the occlusal surface, forming the triangular ridges of the buccal and lingual cusps (Fig 4-37a). The mandibular second premolar has convex triangular ridges.
- Add more wax mesial and distal to the ridges you created to complete the occlusal surface (Fig 4-37b).

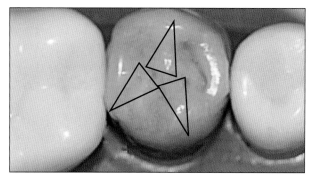

图4-37a 形成三角嵴的加蜡部位（三角形）

Triangles represent where wax is added to form the triangular ridges.

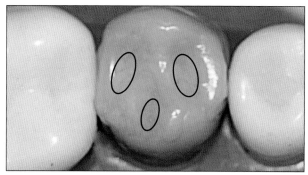

图4-37b 形成𬌗面的加蜡部位（圆形）

Circles represent where wax is filled to complete the occlusal surface.

8. 雕刻𬌗面。

- 首先使用橡子形抛光器标记Y字形沟的位置。Y字形沟由中央沟和舌沟相交而成（图4-38a）。中央沟应与邻牙中央沟成一直线，舌沟延伸至两个舌尖之间

- 使用盘－爪状雕刻刀的小工作尖雕刻锥形的牙尖每个牙尖从牙尖顶向中央沟延伸，从三角嵴向近中边界和远中边界倾斜。下颌第二前磨牙的三角嵴突出

- 按照与相邻边缘嵴相同的高度雕刻边缘嵴。使用Hollenback雕刻刀、盘－爪状雕刻刀来调整边缘嵴的宽度和轮廓。使用尼龙布磨圆、抛光边缘嵴

- 雕刻与对侧同名牙一致的中央沟

- 使用橡子形抛光器或Hollenback雕刻刀的工作尖雕刻三角窝。如果边缘嵴和牙尖堆塑适当，三角窝只需微调即可完成

- 在两个舌尖之间雕刻舌沟，并将其延伸至舌面一小段距离

- 雕刻与对侧同名牙一致的副沟

- 根据需要精修颊楔状隙、舌楔状隙，使其大小和位置与对侧同名牙一致

- 使用注射器吹气或刷子清除𬌗面上多余的蜡屑

- 使用尼龙布抛光𬌗面（图4-38b）

8. Carve the occlusal surface.

- Start by marking the location of the Y-shaped groove with the acorn burnisher. The Y-shaped groove is formed by the intersection of the central and lingual grooves (Fig 4-38a). The central groove should be in line with the central grooves of the adjacent teeth, and the lingual groove extends between the two lingual cusps.

- Use the small discoid-cleoid carver to carve the pyramidal shape of the cusps. Each cusp slopes from the cusp tip to the central groove and from the triangular ridges toward the mesial and distal boundaries. The triangular ridges of the mandibular second premolar are convex.

- Carve the marginal ridges at the same level as the adjacent marginal ridges. Adjust their width and contour with the Hollenback and discoid-cleoid carvers. A nylon stocking is used to round and polish the ridges.

- Carve the central groove identical to that on the contralateral second premolar.

- Carve the triangular fossae with the acorn burnisher or the tip of the Hollenback carver. If you achieve properly contoured marginal ridges and cusps, the triangular fossae are easily emphasized with minimal carving.

- Carve the lingual groove between the two lingual cusps, and extend it onto the lingual surface for a very short distance.

- Carve supplemental grooves identical to those on the contralateral second premolar.

- Refine the buccal and lingual embrasures as needed, so that they are consistent in size and location with those on the contralateral second premolar.

- Remove excess wax flakes on the occlusal surface with an airway syringe or using a brush.

- Polish the occlusal surface with a nylon stocking (Fig 4-38b).

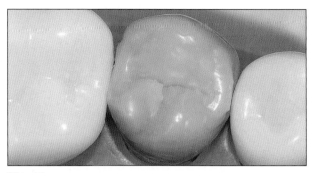

图4-38a

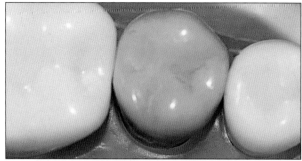

图4-38b

9. 完成最终的雕刻和修形。

- 从不同角度检查线角、点角、楔状隙、邻面接触区、牙尖嵴、殆面解剖结构、外形高点和终止线（图4-39）。根据需要进行加蜡和雕刻，来最终实现蜡型形态与对侧同名牙一致

- 将可摘代模从牙列模型中取出，并与未预备的可摘代模比对。从邻面观来观察牙齿，确保颊面外形高点位于颈1/3处，舌面外形高点位于中1/3处（图4-39e）。确保三角嵴的斜度以及蜡型与终止线平滑过渡。注意牙冠相对于牙根向舌侧倾斜；这是所有下颌后牙的特征（图4-39f）

9. Complete final carving and contouring.

- Line angles, point angles, embrasures, proximal contacts, cusp ridges, occlusal anatomy, heights of contour, and finish line are all checked from different views (Fig 4-39). Wax addition and carving is done as needed to achieve a wax-up that is consistent with the contralateral premolar.

- Remove the tooth from the dentoform. View the tooth from a proximal view to verify that the buccal height of contour is at the cervical third and the lingual height of contour is at the middle third (Fig 4-39e). Notice the convex contour of the triangular ridges. Verify that the wax is in smooth transition with the finish line. Notice the lingual tilt of the crown in relation to the root; this is a feature of all mandibular posterior teeth (Fig 4-39f).

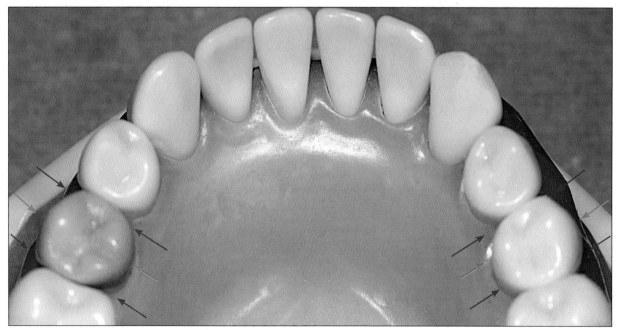

图4-39a　最好从殆面观来观察颊侧线角、舌侧线角（红色箭头）以及颊轴嵴、舌轴嵴（绿色箭头），位置和轮廓应与对侧同名牙一致。颊侧线角和颊轴嵴比舌侧更明显

The buccal and lingual line angles *(red arrows)* and the buccal and lingual ridges *(green arrows)* are best visualized from the occlusal view and should conform in position and contour with those of the contralateral tooth. The buccal line angles and buccal ridge are more prominent than their lingual counterparts.

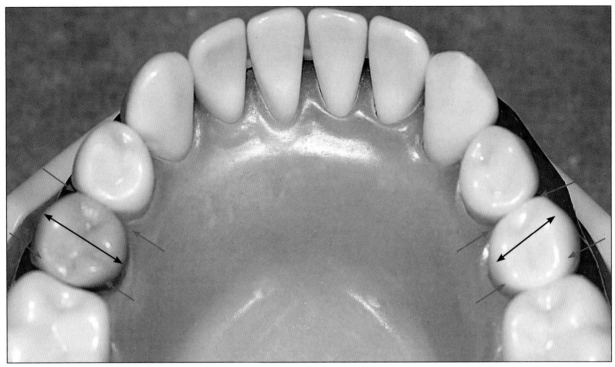

图4-39b 最好从𬌗面观来观察点角（红色箭头），位置和轮廓应与对侧同名牙一致。从𬌗面观来观察时，蜡型的颊舌径（黑色箭头）应该与对侧同名牙一致

The point angles *(red arrows)* are best visualized from the occlusal view and should conform in position and contour to those of the contralateral premolar. The buccolingual dimension of the tooth *(black arrows)* should be identical to the contralateral premolar when viewed occlusally.

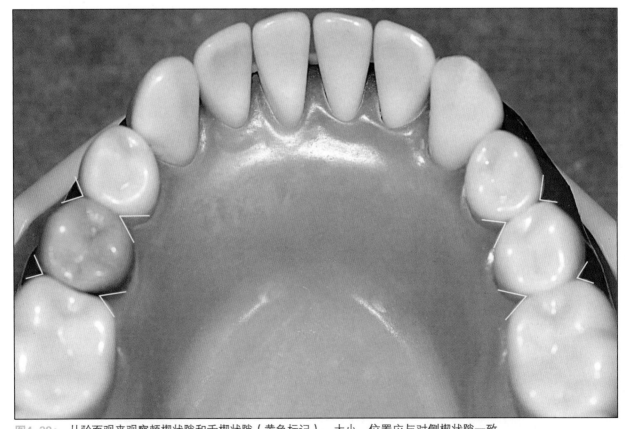

图4-39c 从𬌗面观来观察颊楔状隙和舌楔状隙（黄色标记），大小、位置应与对侧楔状隙一致

The buccal and lingual embrasures *(in yellow)* are visualized from the occlusal view and should match the contralateral embrasures in size and location.

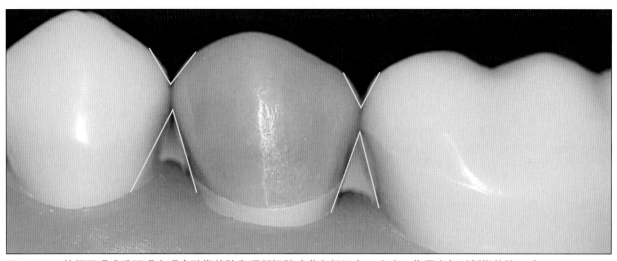

图4-39d 从颊面观或舌面观来观察殆楔状隙和颈邻间隙（黄色标记），大小、位置应与对侧楔状隙一致

Occlusal and cervical embrasures *(in yellow)* are visualized from the buccal or lingual view and should be consistent with the contralateral embrasures.

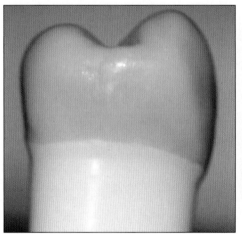

图4-39e 近中邻面观
Mesial view.

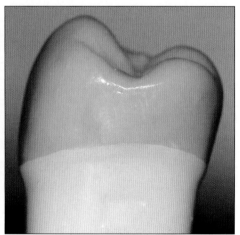

图4-39f 远中邻面观
Distal view.

10. 完成最终的平整和抛光。
- 使用雕刻刀修平表面，使用尼龙布轻轻抛光。这会使蜡型表面高度抛光（图4-40）。应避免长时间抛光，因为可能会改变牙齿的解剖结构。为了避免破坏蜡型，请勿过度加压。使用注射器吹气或刷子清除蜡型和牙列模型上的蜡屑

10. Complete the final smoothing and polishing.
- Plane the surface with a carver and buff lightly with a nylon stocking. This should give your wax-up a nice polished appearance (Fig 4-40). Avoid lengthy polishing as it may change the tooth anatomy, and only use gentle pressure to avoid breaking your wax-up. Remove wax flakes on your wax-up and on the dentoform with the airway syringe or a brush.

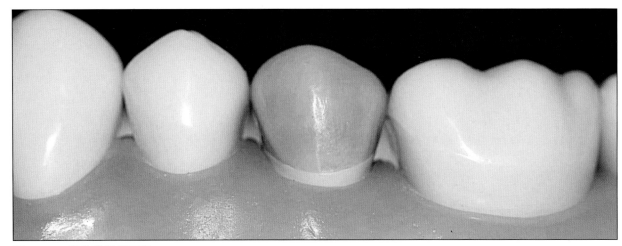

图4-40a　最终蜡型颊面观
Buccal view of final wax-up.

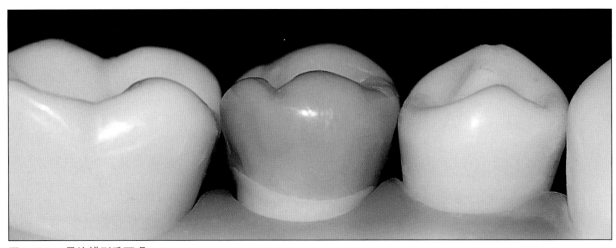

图4-40b　最终蜡型舌面观
Lingual view of final wax-up.

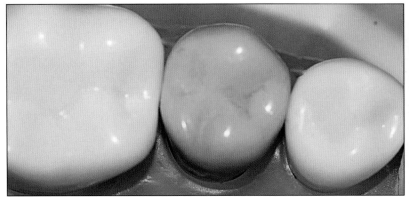

图4-40c

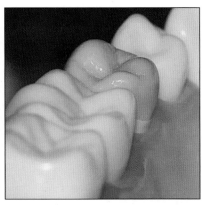

图4-40d

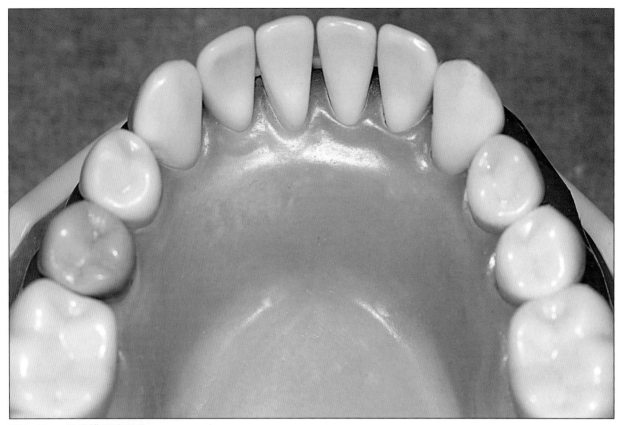

图4-40e 最终蜡型殆面观
Occlusal view of final wax-up.

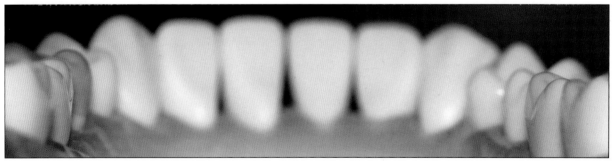

图4-40f 最终蜡型远中邻面观
Distal view of final wax-up.

第5章
Chapter 5

堆塑磨牙蜡型
Waxing Molars

上颌第一磨牙、第二磨牙蜡型堆塑的形态和标准[6-7]

Morphology and Criteria for Maxillary First Molar Wax-Up[6,7]

颊面观

从颊面观可以观察到（图5-1a）：

- 外形呈梯形
- 近中颊尖比远中颊尖宽，但远中颊尖更锐
- 两个颊尖长度近似相等
- 两个颊尖之间有颊发育沟分隔
- 近中接触区位于牙冠𬌗1/3、中1/3交界处
- 远中接触区位于牙冠𬌗颈径和颊舌径的中1/3
- 𬌗楔状隙和颈邻间隙与对侧同名牙一致

舌面观

从舌面观可以观察到（图5-1b）：

- 仅能看到舌尖
- 近中舌尖比远中舌尖大
- 两个舌尖之间有舌发育沟分隔

Buccal view

The following can be observed in the buccal view (Fig 5-1a):

- Geometric outline is trapezoidal.
- Mesiobuccal cusp wider than the distobuccal cusp, but distobuccal cusp more pointed.
- Both cusps nearly the same length.
- Two buccal cusps separated by the buccal developmental groove.
- Mesial contact at the junction of occlusal and middle thirds of the crown.
- Distal contact at the middle third of the crown occlusocervically and buccolingually.
- Occlusal and cervical embrasures consistent with those of the contralateral molar.

Lingual view

The following can be observed in the lingual view (Fig 5-1b):

- Only lingual cusps can be seen.
- Mesiolingual cusp larger than distolingual cusp.
- Two lingual cusps separated by the lingual developmental groove.

- 近中舌尖的舌侧可见卡氏尖
- 舌面光滑凸起
- 𬌗楔状隙和颈邻间隙与对侧同名牙一致

- Carabelli trait seen on the lingual aspect of the mesio-lingual cusp.
- Lingual surface smooth and convex.
- Occlusal and cervical embrasures consistent with those of the contralateral molar.

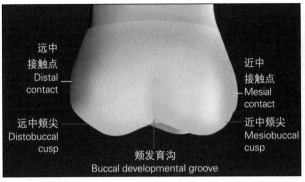

图5-1a

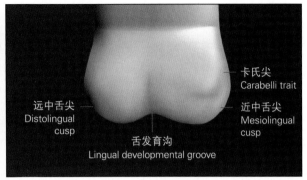

图5-1b

邻面观

从邻面观可以观察到（图5-1c和d）：

- 外形呈梯形
- 颊面外形高点位于颈1/3处
- 舌面外形高点位于中1/3处
- 远中接触区在牙冠𬌗–颈及颊–舌中心

𬌗面观

从𬌗面观可以观察到（图5-1e）：

- 外形呈菱形
- 颊舌径比近远中径大
- 近中颊舌径比远中颊舌径大
- 按牙尖大小排序：近中舌尖>近中颊尖>远中颊尖>远中舌尖>卡氏尖（ML>MB>DB>DL>Carabelli）
- 𬌗面形态由牙尖顶、牙尖嵴、三角嵴、边缘嵴、窝（中央窝、远中窝和两个三角窝）、沟和点隙组成
- 斜嵴是由近中舌尖三角嵴与远中颊尖三角嵴结合而形成的三角嵴。它与边缘嵴处于同一水平，有时也会有发育沟通过

Proximal view

The following can be observed in the proximal views (Figs 5-1c and 5-1d):

- Geometric outline is trapezoidal.
- Buccal height of contour located at the cervical third.
- Lingual height of contour located at the middle third.
- Distal contact area at the center of the crown both cervico-occlusally and buccolingually.

Occlusal view

The following can be observed in the occlusal view (Fig 5-1e):

- Geometric outline is rhomboidal.
- Buccolingual dimension greater than the mesiodistal dimension.
- Buccolingual measurement of the crown greater mesially than distally.
- Cusps in order of size: ML > MB > DB > DL > Carabelli.
- Occlusal morphology includes cusp tips, cusp ridges, triangular ridges, marginal ridges, occlusal fossae (central fossa, distal fossa, and two triangular fossae), grooves, and pits.
- Oblique ridge formed by the union of the triangular ridge of the distobuccal cusp and the distal ridge of the mesiolingual cusp. It is at the same level as the marginal ridges and is sometimes crossed by a developmental groove.

- 线角和点角的位置、轮廓与对侧同名牙一致
- 颊楔状隙和舌楔状隙的大小、位置与对侧同名牙一致

- Line angles and point angles consistent in position and contour to those of the contralateral molar.
- Buccal and lingual embrasures consistent in size and location to those of the contralateral molar.

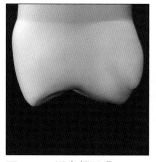

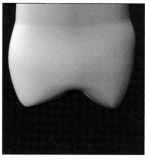

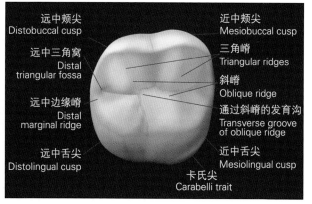

图5-1c　近中邻面观　Mesial view.

图5-1d　远中邻面观　Distal view.

图5-1e

#16MODL（近中–𬌗–远中–舌）嵌体蜡型堆塑步骤

1. 注意可摘代模上牙冠的牙体组织缺损：邻面、部分𬌗面、远中舌尖和部分近中舌尖（图5-2）。
2. 在可摘代模上涂一层初始蜡层，直到覆盖终止线（图5-3）。

Waxing Steps for an MODL Onlay for Tooth #16

1. Notice the missing tooth structure on your tooth peg: proximal surfaces, part of the occlusal surface, the distolingual cusp, and part of the mesiolingual cusp (Fig 5-2).
2. Add an initial layer of wax to cover the finish line on your tooth peg (Fig 5-3).

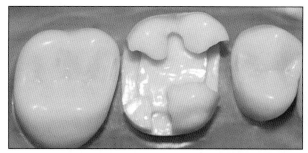

图5-2

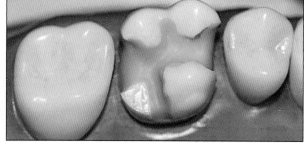

图5-3

3. 以对侧同名牙为参照，在邻牙上标记邻面接触区的位置（图5-4）。
4. 添加蜡锥，将蜡型和邻牙上的标记连接起来（图5-5）。

3. Mark the location of the proximal contacts on the adjacent dentoform teeth. Use the contralateral side as a guide (Fig 5-4).
4. Add wax cones to connect your wax-up to the proximal contacts marked on the adjacent teeth (Fig 5-5).

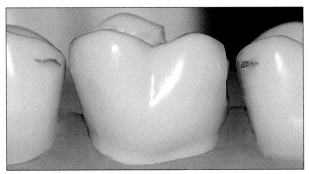

图5-4

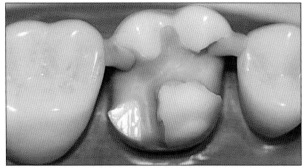

图5-5

5. 添加蜡以形成与邻牙边缘嵴处于同一水平的边缘嵴，然后继续在整个邻面堆蜡（图5-6）。

6. 在牙尖顶对应位置处开始堆蜡以形成远中舌尖（图5-7）。牙尖应该与邻牙牙尖处于同一平面上，并且要比近中舌尖小。

5. Add wax to form the marginal ridges at the same level as the adjacent marginal ridges, and then proceed to wax the entire proximal surface (Fig 5-6).

6. Start building the distolingual cusp by adding wax cones where the tip of the cusp should be located (Fig 5-7). The cusp should be in the same plane as the adjacent cusps and is smaller than the mesiolingual cusp.

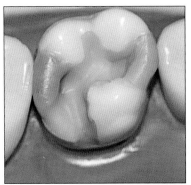

图5-6

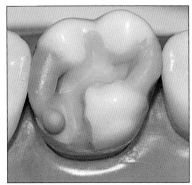

图5-7a

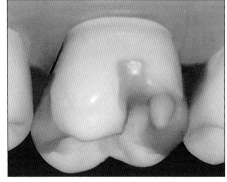

图5-7b

7. 添加蜡以形成远中舌尖的近中牙尖嵴、远中牙尖嵴（图5-8）。

8. 添加蜡以形成近中舌尖的远中牙尖嵴（图5-9）。

7. Add the mesial and distal cusp ridges of the distolingual cusp (Fig 5-8).

8. Add the distal cusp ridge of the mesiolingual cusp (Fig 5-9).

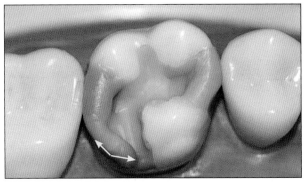

图5-8

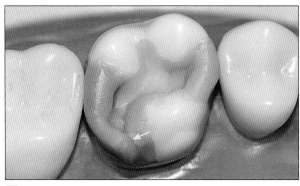

图5-9

9. 添加蜡以形成远中舌尖的三角嵴（图5-10）。
10. 添加蜡以完成牙的舌面（图5-11）。远中舌尖比近中舌尖小且短。

9. Add the triangular ridge of the distolingual cusp (Fig 5-10).
10. Add wax to complete the lingual surface (Fig 5-11). The distolingual cusp is smaller and shorter than the mesiolingual cusp.

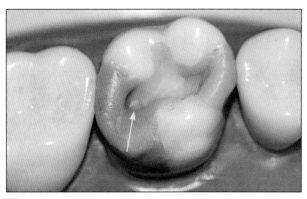

图5-10

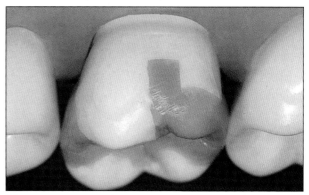

图5-11

11. 完成剩余牙尖的三角嵴。添加更多的蜡以形成连接远中颊尖和近中舌尖的斜嵴。添加蜡以完成骀面的剩余部分（图5-12）。
12. 使用橡子形抛光器和盘-爪状雕刻刀雕刻骀面解剖形态。中央沟与邻牙中央沟成一直线，并且三角嵴应从牙尖顶朝向骀中央倾斜。雕刻的副沟应与对侧同名牙形态相似（图5-13）。

11. Complete the triangular ridges of the remaining cusps. Add more wax to create the oblique ridge that joins the distobuccal and the mesiolingual cusps. Fill in the remainder of the occlusal surface (Fig 5-12).
12. Carve the occlusal anatomy with the acorn burnisher and the small discoid-cleoid carver. The central groove is in line with the central grooves of the adjacent teeth and the triangular ridges should slope from the cusp tips toward the center of the occlusal surface. Carve supplemental grooves similar to the contralateral molar (Fig 5-13).

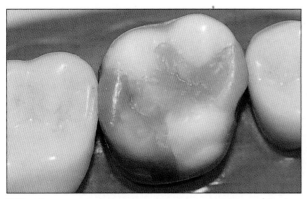

图5-12

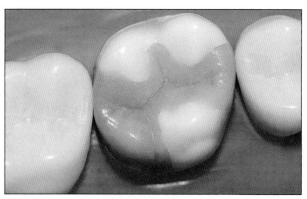

图5-13

13. 平整光滑舌面，然后雕刻分隔两个舌尖的舌发育沟（图5-14）。

14. 从舌面观检查𬌗楔状隙与颈邻间隙（图5-14）。根据需要进行加蜡和雕刻，以使楔状隙与对侧同名牙一致。

15. 从𬌗面观检查颊楔状隙、舌楔状隙（图5-15）。根据需要进行加蜡和雕刻，以使楔状隙与对侧同名牙一致。

13. Plane and smooth the lingual surface, and then carve the lingual developmental groove that separates the two lingual cusps (Fig 5-14).

14. Check the occlusal and cervical embrasures from the lingual view (see Fig 5-14). Wax addition and carving is done as needed to match the embrasures to those of the contralateral molar.

15. Check the buccal and lingual embrasures from the occlusal view (Fig 5-15). Wax addition and carving is done as needed to match the embrasures to those of the contralateral tooth.

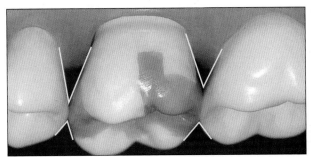

图5-14

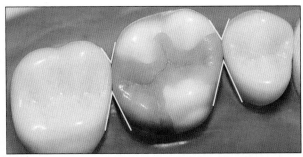

图5-15

16. 使用尼龙布轻轻打磨，平整并抛光蜡型（图5-16）。清除邻牙和牙列模型上的蜡屑。

16. Smooth your wax-up and polish it with a nylon stocking using gentle pressure (Fig 5-16). Remove wax flakes on the adjacent teeth and your dentoform.

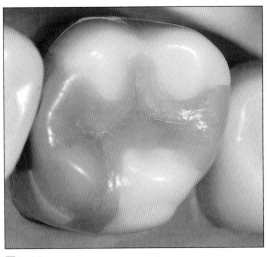

图5-16a

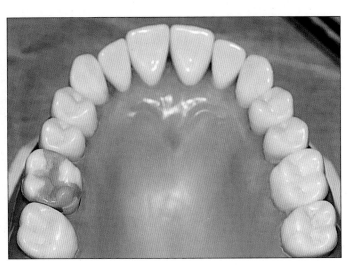

图5-16b

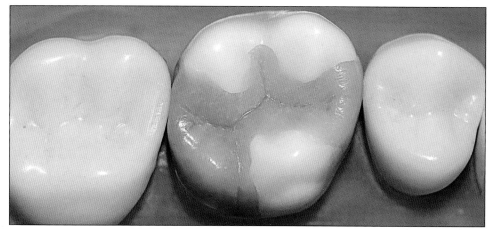

图5-16c　最终蜡型殆面观
Occlusal view of final wax-up.

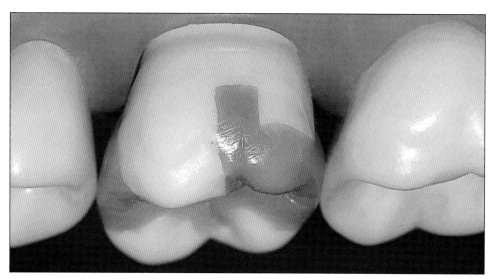

图5-16d　最终蜡型舌面观
Lingual view of final wax-up.

下颌第一磨牙全冠蜡型堆塑的形态和标准[6-7]

颊面观

从颊面观可以观察到（图5-17a）：

- 外形呈梯形
- 5个牙尖都能从颊面观看到
- 因为舌尖比颊尖高，所以在后部可以看到舌尖

Morphology and Criteria for Mandibular First Molar Full-Crown Wax-Up[6,7]

Buccal view

The following can be observed in the buccal view (Fig 5-17a):

- Geometric outline is trapezoidal.
- All the five cusps visible from buccal aspect.
- Lingual cusps seen in the background because they are at a higher level than the buccal cusps.

- 近中颊尖比远中颊尖宽
- 近颊发育沟将两个颊尖分隔
- 远颊发育沟将远中颊尖和远中舌尖分隔
- 近中和远中外形高点位于冠中1/3或殆1/3与中1/3的交界处
- 殆楔状隙和颈邻间隙与对侧同名牙一致

- Mesiobuccal cusp wider than the distobuccal cusp.
- Mesiobuccal developmental groove separates the two buccal cusps.
- Distobuccal developmental groove separates distobuccal and distolingual cusps.
- Mesial and distal heights of contour at the junction of the occlusal and middle thirds or the middle third of the crown.
- Occlusal and cervical embrasures consistent with those of the contralateral molar.

舌面观

从舌面观可以观察到（图5-17b）：

- 外形呈梯形
- 近中舌尖是所有牙尖中最长的
- 舌尖被舌发育沟分隔
- 舌面比颊面窄

Lingual view

The following can be observed in the lingual view (Fig 5-17b):
- Geometric outline is trapezoidal.
- Mesiolingual cusp is the longest of all cusps.
- Lingual cusps separated by the lingual developmental groove.
- Lingual surface narrower than the buccal surface.

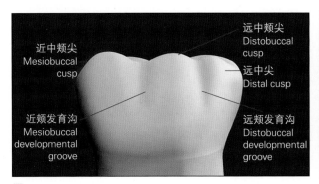

图5-17a

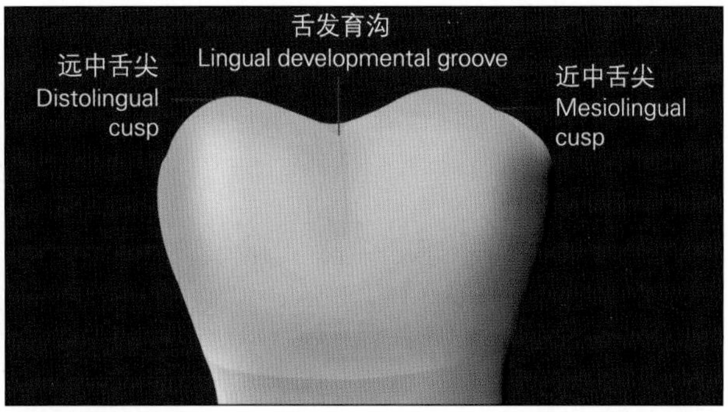

图5-17b

邻面观

从邻面观可以观察到（图5-17c和d）：

- 外形呈菱形
- 牙冠相对于牙根向舌侧倾斜
- 颊面外形高点位于颈1/3处
- 舌面外形高点位于中1/3处
- 颊舌径比近远中径大
- 远中面比近中面短而窄
- 远中边缘嵴比近中边缘嵴短
- 三角嵴从牙尖顶延伸至中央沟

Proximal view

The following can be observed in the proximal views (Figs 5-17c and 5-17d):
- Geometric outline is rhomboidal.
- Crown tilted lingually relative to the root.
- Buccal height of contour at the cervical third.
- Lingual height of contour at the middle third.
- Buccolingual measurement greater on the mesial side than on the distal side.
- Distal surface shorter and narrower than the mesial surface.
- Distal marginal ridge is shorter than the mesial marginal ridge.
- Triangular ridges convex from the cusps tips to the central groove.

殆面观

从殆面观可以观察到（图5-17e）：

- 外形呈五边形
- 近远中径比颊舌径大
- 舌面狭窄（舌向聚合）
- 按牙尖大小排序：近中颊尖＞近中舌尖＞远中舌尖＞远中颊尖＞远中尖（MB＞ML＞DL＞DB＞D）
- 殆面形态由牙尖顶、牙尖嵴、三角嵴、边缘嵴、窝（中央窝和两个三角窝）、沟和点隙组成
- 线角和点角的位置、轮廓与对侧同名牙一致
- 颊楔状隙和舌楔状隙的大小、位置与对侧同名牙一致

Occlusal view

The following can be observed in the occlusal view (Fig 5-17e):

- Geometric outline is pentagonal.
- Mesiodistal measurement greater than the buccolingual measurement.
- Lingual surface narrower (lingual convergence).
- Cusps in order of size: MB > ML > DL > DB > D.
- The occlusal morphology includes cusp tips, cusp ridges, triangular ridges, marginal ridges, occlusal fossae (central fossa and two triangular fossae), grooves, and pits.
- Line angles and point angles consistent in position and contour to those of the contralateral molar.
- Buccal and lingual embrasures consistent in size and location to those of the contralateral molar.

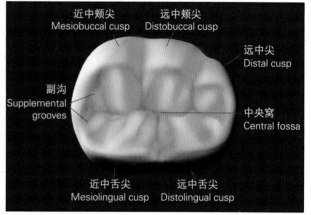

图5-17e

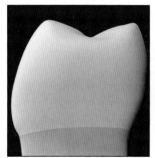

图5-17c　近中邻面观
Mesal view.

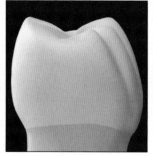

图5-17d　远中邻面观
Distal view.

#36全冠蜡型堆塑步骤

制作全冠蜡型要求更高的精度和对细节的关注，只有这样才能复现其殆面复杂的解剖结构（图5-18）。要注意对侧#46的解剖形态，因为最终完成的#36全冠的各个面应该是对侧#46各个面的镜像。取出#36开始滴蜡堆塑。

1. 形成初始蜡层。

- 手握可摘代模，开始在可摘代模的牙体预备区加蜡。因为下颌第一磨牙是下颌牙弓中最大的牙齿，所以要涂一层较厚的初始蜡层。蜡层厚度均匀，覆盖整个预备区，不留空隙

Waxing Steps for Full-Crown Wax-Up of Tooth #36

Waxing full molars require more precision and attention to detail to create their complex occlusal anatomy (Fig 5-18). Notice the anatomy of the contralateral tooth #46; your final wax-up should be a mirror image of tooth #46 from all views. Unscrew tooth #36 to start your waxing.

1. Establish an initial layer of wax.

- With the tooth peg in your hand, start adding wax to cover the prepared area of the tooth peg. A thicker initial layer of wax is applied because the mandibular first molar is the largest tooth in the mandibular arch. The wax should be even in thickness and have no voids.

- 延长蜡层超过终止线，以确保蜡层边缘没有缺陷
- 使用Hollenback雕刻刀雕刻蜡型，使之与终止线平齐且轮廓合适，以实现与可摘代模的平滑过渡（图5-19）

- Extend the wax past the finish line. This is done to ensure that the wax is not deficient at the margin.
- Use the Hollenback carver to carve the wax flush with the finish line and with the proper contour to achieve a smooth transition with the tooth peg (Fig 5-19).

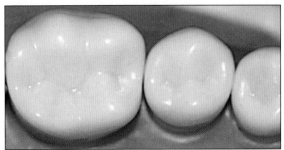 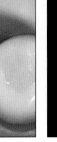 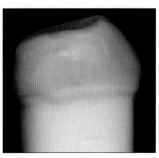

图5-18　　　　　　图5-19a　　　　　　图5-19b

2. 形成邻接关系。
- 在邻牙上标记接触区的位置（图5-20a）。邻面接触区在邻面曲度的最凸处，并且位于牙冠颊舌中心的偏颊侧。模仿对侧同名牙的接触区位置
- 通过在邻面添加蜡锥来形成邻接关系，直到蜡型牢固地与邻牙相接触（图5-20b~d）

2. Establish proximal contacts.
- Mark the location for the proximal contacts on the adjacent teeth (Fig 5-20a). The proximal contacts occur at the crest of curvature of the proximal surfaces and are buccal to the center of the crown buccolingually. Mimic the location of the contacts on the contralateral side.
- Build the proximal contacts by adding wax cones to the proximal surfaces of your wax up until the wax firmly contacts the adjacent teeth (Figs 5-20b to 5-20d).

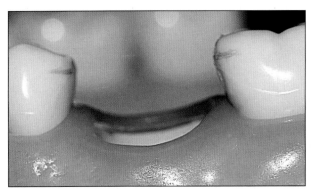 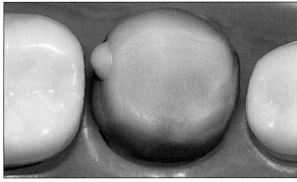

图5-20a　　　　　　图5-20b

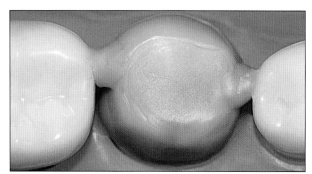

图5-20c 殆面观
Occlusal view.

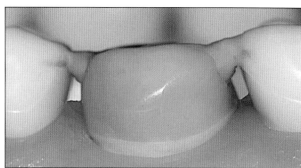

图5-20d 颊面观
Buccal view.

3. 形成邻面接触区。

- 将#36可摘代模从牙列模型中取出，继续在邻面接触区加蜡至龈方终止线，保持蜡表面相对平坦。然后将蜡延伸至覆盖整个邻面（图5-21a）

- 在颊面和舌面涂一层蜡，使可摘代模周围的蜡厚度均匀

- 使用Hollenback雕刻刀清除多余的蜡，并从龈方和颊舌面往接触区方向将邻面雕刻平坦

- 将#36可摘代模放回牙列模型中，并在殆龈向、颊舌向上检查接触区的位置和密合情况（图5-21b~d）

- 在这一步中，可以使用Hollenback雕刻刀清除填塞在颊楔状隙或舌楔状隙的多余的蜡

3. Wax the proximal surface.

- Remove the tooth #36 from the dentoform and add wax to join the waxed proximal contact to the gingival finish line, keeping the wax relatively flat. Then extend the wax to cover the entire proximal surface (Fig 5-21a).

- Apply a layer of wax to the buccal and lingual surfaces to make the thickness of the wax even around the tooth peg.

- Use the Hollenback carver to remove excess wax and carve the proximal surfaces flat cervical to the contact and buccolingually.

- Return the tooth #36 to the dentoform and verify the location and closure of the proximal contacts in the occlusogingival and buccolingual directions (Figs 5-21b to 5-21d).

- Excess wax blocking the buccal or lingual embrasures can be carved at this step with the Hollenback carver.

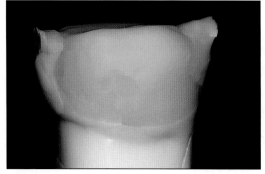

图5-21a

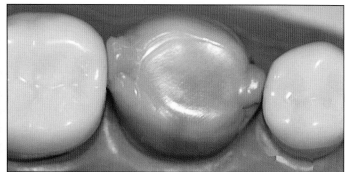

图5-21b 殆面观
Occlusal view.

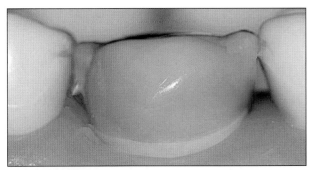

图5-21c　颊面观
Buccal view.

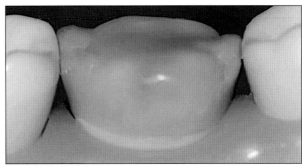

图5-21d　舌面观
Lingual view.

4. 形成𬌗面边界。

- 形成牙尖顶。保持可摘代模在牙列模型中，在颊尖、舌尖对应位置添加蜡锥，并使其高度合适（图5-22a和b）。**位置**：牙尖应该与邻牙牙尖在同一平面上。**高度**：舌尖比颊尖高

- 按牙尖高度排序：近中舌尖>远中舌尖>近中颊尖>远中颊尖>远中尖（ML>DL>MB>DB>D）

- 按牙尖大小排序：近中颊尖>近中舌尖>远中舌尖>远中颊尖>远中尖（MB>ML>DL>DB>D）

- 形成牙尖嵴。加蜡以形成颊尖及舌尖的近中、远中牙尖嵴（图5-22c和d）。从牙尖顶向近中和远中倾斜形成𬌗面边界。边缘嵴堆蜡可以在此步骤进行，或也可以在颊面、舌面堆蜡后。然而，对于磨牙来说，在完成颊面、舌面轮廓后，可能更容易给边缘嵴加蜡

4. Wax the boundaries of the occlusal surface.

- Form the cusp tips. With the tooth in the dentoform, add wax cones to place the buccal and lingual cusp tips at their proper location and with the approximate proper height (Figs 5-22a and 5-22b). **Location:** The cusp tips should be in the same plane as those of the adjacent teeth. **Height:** The lingual cusps are higher than the buccal cusps.

- Cusps in order of height: ML > DL > MB > DB > D.

- Cusps in order of size: MB > ML > DL > DB > D.

- Establish the cusp ridges. Add wax to establish the mesial and distal cusp ridges of the buccal and lingual cusps (Figs 5-22c and 5-22d). These slope from the cusp tip mesially and distally to form the boundaries of the occlusal surface. Marginal ridges may be waxed at this step or after waxing the buccal and lingual surfaces. However, for molars it may be easier to wax the marginal ridges after completing the buccal and lingual contours.

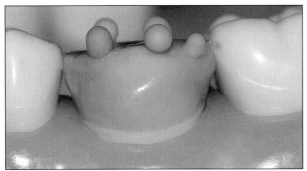

图5-22a　颊面观
Buccal view.

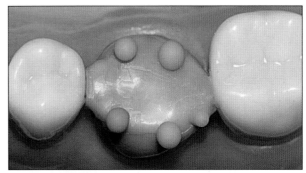

图5-22b　𬌗面观
Occlusal view.

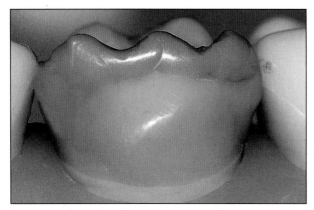

图5-22c　颊面观
Buccal view.

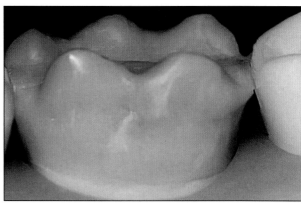

图5-22d　舌面观
Lingual view.

5. 堆塑颊面。

• 在颊面加蜡，完成颊面轮廓（图5-23a）。在颈1/3处添加更多的蜡，形成外形高点。然后通过将颊面外形高点的近中边界和远中边界与相应的牙尖嵴相连而形成线角。保持可摘代模在牙列模型中，添加颊面轮廓，以实现精确定位

• 使用堆蜡工具在剩余区域加蜡。这可以通过将可摘代模放回牙列模型中或从牙列模型中取出可摘代模来完成

• 清除多余的蜡以获得光滑的颊面，使线角、外形高点保持位置和轮廓适当

• 雕刻形成近颊、远颊发育沟（图5-23b）

5. Wax the buccal surface.

• Add wax to the buccal surface to complete the buccal contour (Fig 5-23a). More wax is applied at the cervical third to form the height of contour. The line angles are then waxed by joining the mesial and distal ends of the buccal height of contour to the corresponding cusp ridges. The contours are added with the tooth in the dentoform for precise localization.

• Fill in the remaining areas with wax using your wax-addition instruments. This can be done with the tooth inside or outside of the dentoform.

• Carve the excess wax to achieve a smooth buccal surface, maintaining the proper position and contour of the line angles and height of contour.

• Carve the mesiobuccal and distobuccal developmental grooves (Fig 5-23b).

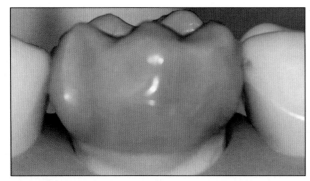

图5-23a

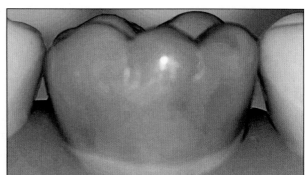

图5-23b

6. 堆塑舌面。

- 舌面加蜡，完成舌面轮廓（图5-24a）。添加更多的蜡，形成舌面外形高点。然后通过将舌面外形高点的近中边界和远中边界与相应的牙尖嵴相连而形成线角。舌侧线角不如颊侧线角明显，整个舌面相当突出

- 在剩余区域加蜡

- 清除多余的蜡以获得光滑的舌面，使线角、外形高点保持位置和轮廓适当

- 在舌尖之间雕刻形成舌发育沟（图5-24b）

6. Wax the lingual surface.

- Add wax to the lingual surface to complete the lingual contour (Fig 5-24a). More wax is applied at the middle third to form the height of contour. The line angles are then waxed by joining the mesial and distal ends of the lingual height of contour to the corresponding cusp ridges. The lingual line angles are less prominent than the buccal line angles and the entire lingual surface is quite convex.
- Fill in the remaining areas with wax.
- Carve the excess wax to achieve a smooth lingual surface, maintaining the proper position and contour of the line angles and height of contour.
- Carve the lingual developmental groove between the lingual cusps (Fig 5-24b).

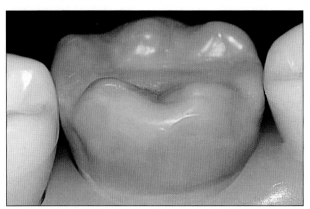

图5-24a

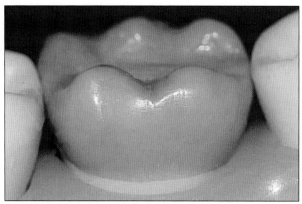

图5-24b

7. 形成边缘嵴、三角嵴和完成𬌗面。

- 形成边缘嵴。加蜡，形成边缘嵴。这一步将完成𬌗面的轮廓（图5-25a）

- 形成三角嵴。加蜡将牙尖顶连接到𬌗面的中心，形成颊尖和舌尖的三角嵴（图5-25b）

- 加蜡，填充𬌗面的剩余部分（图5-25c）。这一步操作非常精细，需要使用PKT2雕刻刀的末端

7. Establish the marginal and triangular ridges and complete the occlusal surface.

- Establish the marginal ridges. Add wax to establish the marginal ridges. This will complete the outline of the occlusal surface (Fig 5-25a).
- Establish the triangular ridges. Apply wax to connect the cusp tips to the center of the occlusal surface forming the triangular ridges of the buccal and lingual cusps (Fig 5-25b).
- Add wax to fill in the rest of the occlusal surface (Fig 5-25c). For this very delicate step, use the end of the PKT2 instrument.

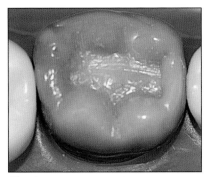

图5-25a

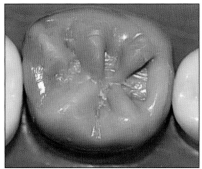

图5-25b

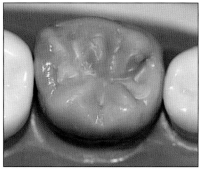

图5-25c

8. 雕刻殆面。

- 首先使用橡子形抛光器标记中央沟的位置，中央沟应与邻牙中央沟成一直线（图5-26a）
- 使用盘-爪状雕刻刀的小工作尖雕刻锥形的牙尖。每个牙尖从牙尖顶向中央沟延伸，从三角嵴向近中边界和远中边界倾斜
- 雕刻与对侧同名牙一致的中央沟和副沟
- 按照与相邻边缘嵴相同的高度雕刻边缘嵴。使用Hollenback雕刻刀、盘-爪状雕刻刀来调整边缘嵴的宽度和轮廓。使用尼龙布磨圆、抛光边缘嵴
- 使用橡子形抛光器或Hollenback雕刻刀的工作尖雕刻三角窝
- 在颊尖之间雕刻近中颊沟和远中颊沟
- 在两个舌尖之间雕刻舌沟
- 根据需要精修颊楔状隙、舌楔状隙
- 使用注射器吹气或刷子清除殆面上多余的蜡屑
- 使用尼龙布抛光殆面（图5-26b）

8. Carve the occlusal surface.

- Start with marking the location of the central groove with the acorn burnisher, the central groove should be in line with the central grooves of the adjacent teeth (Fig 5-26a).
- Use the small discoid-cleoid carver to carve the pyramidal shape of the cusps. Each cusp slopes from cusp tip to the central groove and from the triangular ridges toward the mesial and distal boundaries.
- Carve the central groove and the supplemental grooves identical to the contralateral tooth.
- Carve the marginal ridges at the same level as the adjacent marginal ridges. Adjust the width and contour of the marginal ridges with the Hollenback and discoid-cleoid carvers. A nylon stocking is used to round and polish the ridges.
- Carve the triangular fossae with the acorn burnisher or the tip of the Hollenback carver.
- Carve the mesiobuccal and distobuccal grooves between the buccal cusps.
- Carve the lingual groove between the two lingual cusps.
- Refine the buccal and lingual embrasures as needed.
- Remove excess wax flakes on the occlusal surface with the airway syringe or using a brush.
- Polish the occlusal surface with a nylon stocking (Fig 5-26b).

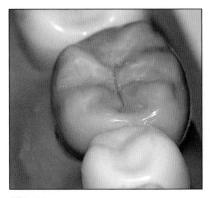

图5-26a

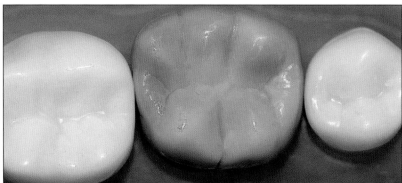

图5-26b　殆面（最终雕刻面）

Final carving of the occlusal surface.

9. 完成最终的雕刻和修形。

• 从不同角度检查线角、点角、楔状隙、邻面接触区、牙尖嵴、𬌗面解剖结构、外形高点和终止线（图5-27）。根据需要进行加蜡和雕刻，来最终实现蜡型形态与对侧同名牙一致

9. Complete final carving and contouring.

• Line angles, point angles, embrasures, proximal contacts, cusp ridges, occlusal anatomy, heights of contours, and finish line are all checked from different views (Fig 5-27). Wax addition and carving is done as needed to achieve a wax-up that is consistent with the contralateral molar.

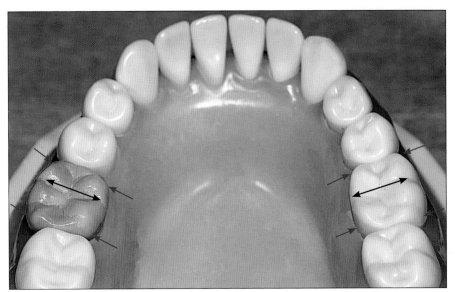

图5-27a　最好从𬌗面观来观察颊侧线角、舌侧线角及点角（红色箭头），位置和轮廓应与对侧同名牙一致。颊侧线角和点角比舌侧更明显。从𬌗面观来观察时，蜡型的颊舌径（黑色箭头）应该与对侧同名牙一致

Buccal and lingual line and point angles *(red arrows)* are best visualized from occlusal view and should conform in position and contour with those of the contralateral molar. The buccal line angles and point angles are more prominent than their lingual counterparts. The buccolingual dimension of the tooth *(black arrows)* should be identical to the contralateral first molar when viewed occlusally.

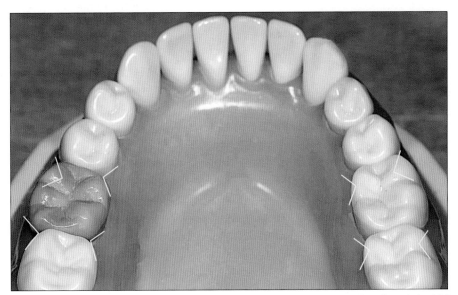

图5-27b　从𬌗面观来观察颊楔状隙和舌楔状隙（黄色标记），大小、位置应与对侧楔状隙一致

The buccal and lingual embrasures *(in yellow)* are visualized from the occlusal view and should match the contralateral embrasures in size and location.

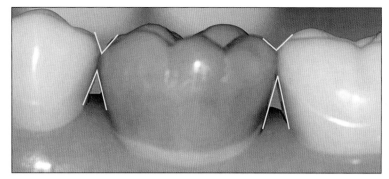

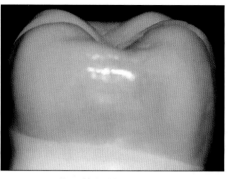

图5-27c 从颊面观或舌面观来观察殆楔状隙和颈邻间隙（黄色标记），大小、位置应与对侧楔状隙一致

Occlusal and cervical embrasures *(in yellow)* are visualized from a buccal or lingual view and should be consistent with the contralateral embrasures.

图5-27d 将可摘代模从牙列模型中取出。从邻面观来观察蜡型，确保颊面外形高点位于颈1/3，舌面外形高点位于中1/3，蜡型的终止线与可摘代模平滑过渡

Remove the tooth from the dentoform. View the tooth from a proximal view to verify that the buccal height of contour is at the cervical third, the lingual height of contour is at the middle third, and the wax is in smooth transition with the finish line.

10. 完成最终的平整和抛光。

• 使用雕刻刀修平表面，使用尼龙布轻轻抛光。这会使蜡型表面高度抛光（图5-28）。应避免长时间抛光，因为这样可能会改变牙齿的解剖结构。为了避免破坏蜡型，请勿过度加压。使用注射器吹气或刷子清除蜡型和牙列模型上的蜡屑

10. Complete final smoothing and polishing.

• Plane the surface with a carver, and buff lightly with a nylon stocking. This should give your wax-up a nice polished appearance (Fig 5-28). Avoid lengthy polishing because it may change the tooth anatomy, and use only gentle pressure to avoid breaking your wax-up. Remove wax flakes on your wax-up and on the dentoform with the airway syringe or a brush.

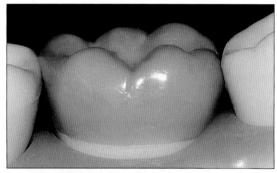

图5-28a 最终蜡型舌面观
Lingual view of final wax-up.

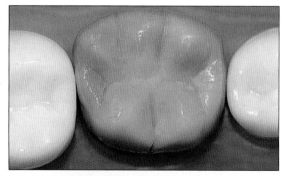

图5-28b 最终蜡型殆面观
Occlusal view of final wax-up.

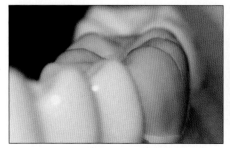

图5-28c 最终蜡型近中邻面观
Mesial view of final wax-up.

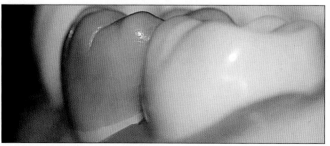

图5-28d 最终蜡型远中邻面观
Distal view of final wax-up.

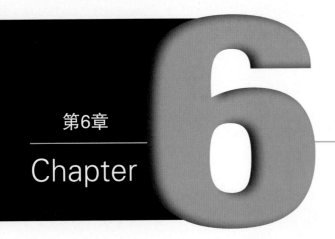

第6章

Chapter

全冠蜡型的评价说明
Evaluation Criteria for Full-Crown Wax-Ups

一般标准

- 蜡型是对侧同名牙在各个面的镜像：唇/颊面、舌面、殆/切面和邻面等。唯一的例外是邻接，即使对侧同名牙没有邻接，蜡型也应该有邻接

- 精确复制外形高点、线角和点角，实现与对侧同名牙一致、与邻牙和谐

- 精确复制所有的解剖标志——包括窝、沟、嵴、舌隆突

- 近中接触区在唇舌向/颊舌向、殆颈向位置均适当

- 与相邻的边缘嵴高度相同

- 精确复制楔状隙的大小和位置，与对侧同名牙一致

- 蜡型光滑，没有流线、划痕和异物

- 蜡与预备好的可摘代模融合在一起，不会超出预备好的终止线

- 可摘代模和牙列模型的其余部分没有蜡屑

- 蜡完全覆盖可摘代模，颜色和厚度均匀

General Criteria

- The wax-up is a mirror image of the contralateral tooth from all views: facial, lingual, occlusal/incisal, and proximal. The only exception is the proximal contact, which should be closed even if the contact on the contralateral side is open.

- Heights of contour, line angles, and point angles are duplicated precisely to match those of the contralateral tooth and achieve harmony with the adjacent teeth.

- All anatomical landmarks—including fossae, grooves, ridges, and cingulae—are duplicated precisely.

- Proximal contacts are at the proper location facio-lingually and occlusocervically.

- Adjacent marginal ridges are at the same height.

- Embrasure size and location are duplicated precisely to match those of the contralateral tooth.

- The wax-up is smooth and free of flow lines, scratches, and foreign substance.

- The wax is confluent with the prepared tooth peg and does not extend beyond the prepared finish line.

- The remainder of the tooth peg and the dentoform are free of wax and debris.

- The wax completely covers the tooth peg and has a uniform color and thickness.

评价说明

- 评价说明分为4个部分
- 相似的标准和相互依赖的标准大多放在同一节中。例如,邻接,如果放错位置,将导致楔状隙的大小不正确
- 每项评价标准都属于以下三类之一
  - **高水平**的性能,**>90%**的准确率(即不需要更正)
  - **中水平**的性能,**80%~90%**的准确率(即需要最少的修正)
  - **低水平**的性能,**<80%**的准确率(即需要大量修正)
- 正确地复制解剖形态和轮廓,并制作出高度平滑和完整的蜡型是一年级牙科学生的最终目标。制作精美的蜡型和艺术品是非常受欢迎的和渴望的。然而,不要忘记,堆蜡的全部目的是为了学习牙齿解剖和获得动手技能

前牙蜡型的评价说明

见表6-1~表6-4。

Evaluation Rubric

- The evaluation rubric is divided into four sections.
- Similar criteria and those that are dependent on each other are mostly placed in the same section. For example, proximal contacts, if misplaced, will result in improper size of embrasures.
- Each criteria evaluated falls into one of three categories;
  - **High level** of performance, **> 90%** accuracy (ie, no corrections are needed)
  - **Moderate level** of performance, ranging from **80% to 90%** accuracy (ie, minimal corrections are needed)
  - **Low level** of performance, **< 80%** accuracy (ie, major corrections are needed)
- Properly duplicating anatomy and contours and producing a highly smooth and finished wax-up is the ultimate goal for first-year dental students. Producing a beautiful wax-up and a work of art is highly appreciated and desired. However, it should not be forgotten that the whole purpose of waxing is to learn tooth anatomy and acquire hand skills.

Evaluation Rubric for Anterior Wax-Ups

See Table 6-1 to Table 6-4.

表6-1 邻接、邻面轮廓、楔状隙

	高性能	中性能	低性能
邻接	近中和远中接触区位置、大小正确	位置和/或大小有微小差异	位置和/或大小存在重大差异
邻面轮廓	近中面和远中面轮廓适当	略凸/略凹	过凸/过凹
楔状隙	位置、大小与对侧同名牙一致	• 略小/略大 • 略有错位	• 过小/过大 • 过度错位

Table 6-1 Proximal contacts, proximal contours, and embrasures

	High performance	Moderate performance	Low performance
Proximal contacts	Mesial and distal contacts have correct position and size	Minor discrepancy in position and/or size	Major discrepancy in position and/or size
Proximal contours	Mesial and distal surfaces have proper contour	Slightly convex/concave	Excessively convex/concave
Embrasures	Consistent with those of the contralateral tooth in location and size	• Slightly small/large • Slight malposition	• Excessively small/large • Excessive malposition

表6-2 线角、点角和切缘

	高性能	中性能	低性能
线角	位置和轮廓与对侧同名牙一致	• 略有错位 • 略微锋利/略微圆钝	• 过度错位 • 过于锋利/过于圆钝
点角	位置和轮廓与对侧同名牙一致	• 略有错位 • 略微锋利/略微圆钝	• 过度错位 • 过于锋利/过于圆钝
切缘			
宽度	宽度适当	略宽/略窄	过宽/过窄
外形和斜度	外形和斜度适当	• 略凸/略凹 • 斜度不适当	• 过凸/过凹 • 过度倾斜
位置	唇舌和切龈位置（牙冠长度）适当	略有错位	过度错位
厚度	厚度适当	略厚/略薄	过厚/过薄

Table 6-2 Line angles, point angles, and incisal edge

	High performance	Moderate performance	Low performance
Line angles	Consistent with those of the contralateral tooth in position and contour	• Slight malposition • Slightly sharp/rounded	• Excessive malposition • Excessively sharp/rounded
Point angles	Consistent with those of the contralateral tooth in position and contour	• Slight malposition • Slightly sharp/rounded	• Excessive malposition • Excessively sharp/rounded
Incisal edge			
Width	Proper width	Slightly wide/narrow	Excessively wide/narrow
Shape and slope	Proper shape and slope	• Slightly convex/concave • Improper slope	• Excessively convex/concave • Excessive slope
Position	Proper labiolingual and incisogingival position (tooth length)	Slight malposition	Excessive malposition
Thickness	Proper thickness	Slightly thick/thin	Excessively thick/thin

表6-3 唇面轮廓、舌面轮廓和舌面解剖结构

	高性能	中性能	低性能
唇面轮廓	• 唇面轮廓适当 • 外形高点位置适当	• 略凸/略凹 • 外形高点略有错位 • 唇舌径略厚/略薄	• 过凸/过凹 • 外形高点过度错位 • 唇舌径过大
舌面轮廓	• 舌面轮廓适当 • 外形高点位置适当	• 略凸/略凹 • 外形高点略有错位	• 过凸/过凹 • 外形高点过度错位
舌面解剖结构			
舌隆突	位置和轮廓适当	• 略有错位 • 略平坦/略大	• 过度错位 • 过于平坦/过大
舌窝	宽度和深度适当	• 略宽/略窄 • 略浅/略深	• 过宽/过窄 • 过浅/过深
边缘嵴	与相邻边缘嵴宽度和高度相当	• 略宽/略窄 • 略高/略低	• 过宽/过窄 • 过高/过低

Table 6-3 Labial contour, lingual contour, and lingual anatomy

	High performance	Moderate performance	Low performance
Labial contour	• Proper contour of labial surface • Height of contour at proper location	• Slightly convex/concave • Slight malposition in height of contour • Labiolingual dimension is slightly thick/thin	• Excessively convex/concave • Excessive malposition in height of contour • Excessive labiolingual dimension
Lingual contour	• Proper contour of lingual surface • Height of contour at proper location	• Slightly convex/concave • Slight malposition in height of contour	• Excessively convex/concave • Excessive malposition in height of contour
Lingual anatomy			
Cingulum	Proper position and contour	• Slight malposition • Slightly flat/bulky	• Excessive malposition • Excessively flat/bulky
Lingual fossa	Proper width and depth	• Slightly wide/narrow • Slightly shallow/deep	• Excessively wide/narrow • Excessively shallow/deep
Marginal ridges	Proper width and level with the adjacent ridges	• Slightly wide/narrow • Slightly high/low	• Excessively wide/narrow • Excessively high/low

表6-4 边缘完整性、表面光洁度和整洁

	高性能	中性能	低性能
边缘完整性	• 蜡轮廓边缘适当 • 蜡恰好在边缘终止	• 边缘外形突度略大/略小 • 边缘略微过长/略微过短	• 边缘外形突度过大/过小 • 边缘过长/过短
表面光洁度	• 蜡表面光滑，无流线和划痕 • 高度抛光	• 有一些划痕或流线 • 略钝	• 严重凹陷和划痕 • 表面过于暗淡、凹凸不平和不规则 • 抛光不足
整洁	• 牙列模型上没有蜡屑 • 蜡型上或蜡型中没有异物	• 牙列模型上有少量蜡屑 • 蜡型上或蜡型内有极少量异物	• 牙列模型上有许多蜡屑 • 蜡型上或蜡型内有大量异物

Table 6-4 Marginal integrity, surface finish and neatness

	High performance	Moderate performance	Low performance
Marginal integrity	• Proper wax contour at the margin • Wax terminated precisely at the margin	• Slightly over-/undercontoured at the margin • Slightly overextended/deficient at the margin	• Excessively over-/undercontoured at the margin • Excessively overextended/deficient at the margin
Surface finish	• Smooth surface of wax free of flow lines and scratches • Nicely polished	• A few scratches or flow lines • Slightly dull	• Major depressions and scratches • Excessively dull, pitted, and irregular surface • Lack of polish
Neatness	• No wax flakes on the dentoform • No foreign substance on or embedded in the wax-up	• A few wax flakes on the dentoform • Minimal amount of foreign substance on or embedded in the wax-up	• Many wax flakes on the dentoform • Substantial amount of foreign substance on or embedded in the wax-up

后牙蜡型的评价说明

见表6-5~表6-8。

Evaluation Rubric for Posterior Wax-Ups

See Table 6-5 to Table 6-8.

表6-5 邻接、邻面外形、楔状隙和整洁

	高性能	中性能	低性能
邻接	近中和远中接触区位置、大小正确	位置和/或大小有微小差异	位置和/或大小存在重大差异
邻面外形	近中面和远中面外形适当	略凸/略凹	过凸/过凹
楔状隙	位置、大小与对侧同名牙一致	• 略小/略大 • 略有错位	• 过小/过大 • 过度错位
整洁	• 牙列模型上没有蜡屑 • 蜡型上或蜡型中没有异物	• 牙列模型上有少量蜡屑 • 蜡型上或蜡型内有极少量异物	• 牙列模型上有许多蜡屑 • 蜡型上或蜡型内有大量异物

Table 6-5 Proximal contacts, contours, embrasures and neatness

	High performance	Moderate performance	Low performance
Proximal contacts	Mesial and distal contacts have correct position and size	Minor discrepancy in position and/or size	Major discrepancy in position and/or size
Proximal contours	Mesial and distal surfaces have proper contour	Slightly convex/concave	Excessively convex/concave
Embrasures	Consistent with those of the contralateral tooth in location and size	• Slightly small/large • Slight malposition	• Excessively small/large • Excessive malposition
Neatness	• No wax flakes on the dentoform • No foreign substance on or embedded in the wax-up	• A few wax flakes on the dentoform • Minimal amount of foreign substance on or embedded in the wax-up	• Many wax flakes on the dentoform • Substantial amount of foreign substance on or embedded in the wax-up

表6-6　线角、点角和边缘完整性

	高性能	中性能	低性能
线角	位置和轮廓与对侧同名牙一致	• 略有错位 • 略微锋利/略微圆钝	• 过度错位 • 过于锋利/过于圆钝
点角	位置和轮廓与对侧同名牙一致	• 略有错位 • 略微锋利/略微圆钝	• 过度错位 • 过于锋利/过于圆钝
边缘完整性	• 蜡轮廓边缘适当 • 蜡恰好在边缘终止	• 边缘外形突度略大/略小 • 边缘略微过长/略微过短	• 边缘外形突度过大/过小 • 边缘过长/过短

Table 6-6 Line angles, point angles, and marginal integrity

	High performance	Moderate performance	Low performance
Line angles	Consistent with those of the contralateral tooth in position and contour	• Slight malposition • Slightly sharp/rounded	• Excessive malposition • Excessively sharp/rounded
Point angles	Consistent with those of the contralateral tooth in position and contour	• Slight malposition • Slightly sharp/rounded	• Excessive malposition • Excessively sharp/rounded
Marginal integrity	• Proper wax contour at the margin • Wax terminated precisely at margin	• Slightly over-/undercontoured at the margin • Slightly overextended/ deficient at the margin	• Excessively over-/ undercontoured at the margin • Excessively overextended/ deficient at the margin

表6-7 颊面轮廓、舌面轮廓和表面光洁度

	高性能	中性能	低性能
颊面轮廓	• 突度正常 • 外形高点位置适当 • 颊舌径适当	• 略凸/略凹 • 外形高点略有错位 • 颊舌径略厚/略薄	• 过凸/过凹 • 外形高点过度错位 • 颊舌径过大
舌面轮廓	• 突度正常 • 外形高点位置适当	• 略凸/略凹 • 外形高点略有错位	• 过凸/过凹 • 外形高点过度错位
表面光洁度	• 蜡表面光滑，无流线和划痕 • 高度抛光	• 有一些划痕或流线 • 略钝	• 严重凹陷和划痕 • 表面过于暗淡、凹凸不平和不规则 • 抛光不足

Table 6-7 Buccal and lingual contours and surface finish

	High performance	Moderate performance	Low performance
Buccal contour	• Proper contour • Height of contour at proper location • Proper buccolingual dimension	• Slightly convex/concave • Slight malposition in height of contour • Buccolingual thickness is slightly thick/thin	• Excessively convex/concave • Excessive malposition in height of contour • Excessive buccolingual dimension
Lingual contour	• Proper contour of lingual surface • Height of contour at proper location	• Slightly convex/concave • Slight malposition in height of contour	• Excessively convex/concave • Excessive malposition in height of contour
Surface finish	• Smooth surface of wax, free of flow lines and scratches • Nicely polished	• A few scratches or flow lines • slightly dull	• Major depressions and scratches • Excessively dull, pitted, and irregular • Lack of polish

表6-8 **殆面解剖结构**

	高性能	中性能	低性能
牙尖	高度、位置、形状及大小适当	• 略有错位 • 略大/略小 • 牙尖顶略微过于锋利/过于圆钝	• 过度错位 • 过大/小 • 牙尖顶过于锋利/过于圆钝
边缘嵴	与相邻边缘嵴宽度和高度相当	• 略宽/略窄 • 略高/略低	• 过宽/过窄 • 过高/过低
三角嵴和牙尖嵴	突度和斜度适当	• 外形突度略大/略小 • 斜度略浅/略陡	• 外形突度过大/过小 • 斜度过浅/过陡
沟	位置和清晰度适当	• 略有错位 • 略深/略浅	• 过度错位 • 过深/过浅
窝	位置、深度和宽度适当	• 略有错位 • 略深/略浅 • 略宽/略窄	• 过度错位 • 过深/过浅 • 过宽/过窄

Table 6-8 **Occlusal morphology**

	High performance	Moderate performance	Low performance
Cusps	Proper height, position, shape, and size	• Slight malposition • Slightly large/small • Cusp tips slightly too sharp/rounded	• Excessive malposition • Excessively large/small • Cusp tips excessively sharp/rounded
Marginal ridges	Proper width and height, level with adjacent ridges	• Slightly wide/narrow • Slightly high/low	• Excessively wide/narrow • Excessively high/low
Triangular ridges and cusp ridges	Proper contour and slope	• Slightly over-/undercontoured • Slightly shallow or steep slope	• Excessively over-/undercontoured • Excessively shallow or too steep of slope
Grooves	Proper position and definition	• Slight malposition • Slightly shallow/deep	• Excessive malposition • Excessively shallow/deep
Fossae	Proper location, depth, and width	• Slight malposition • Slightly shallow/deep • Slightly wide/narrow	• Excessive malposition • Excessively shallow/deep • Excessively wide/narrow

图文编辑

刘 菲 刘 娜 康 鹤 肖 艳 王静雅 纪凤薇 刘玉卿 张 浩 曹 勇 杨 洋

This is a translation edition of Waxing for Dental Students, by Rowida Abdalla, published by arrangement with Quintessence Publishing Co., Inc.

© 2018 Quintessence Publishing Co., Inc.

©2023，辽宁科学技术出版社。
著作权合同登记号：06–2021第152号。

图书在版编目（CIP）数据

蜡型堆塑教程 /（埃及）罗维达·阿布达拉（Rowida Abdalla）
编著；赵今，林静主译.—沈阳：辽宁科学技术出版社，2023.10
ISBN 978-7-5591-2368-8

Ⅰ.①蜡… Ⅱ.①罗… ②赵… ③林… Ⅲ.①口腔科学—
教材 Ⅳ.①R78

中国版本图书馆CIP数据核字（2021）第265946号

出版发行：辽宁科学技术出版社
　　　　　（地址：沈阳市和平区十一纬路25号　邮编：110003）
印 刷 者：深圳市福圣印刷有限公司
经 销 者：各地新华书店
幅面尺寸：210mm×285mm
印　　张：8
插　　页：4
字　　数：165千字
出版时间：2023年10月第1版
印刷时间：2023年10月第1次印刷
策划编辑：陈　刚
责任编辑：金　烁
封面设计：袁　舒
版式设计：袁　舒
责任校对：李　霞

书　　号：ISBN 978-7-5591-2368-8
定　　价：98.00元

投稿热线：024-23280336
邮购热线：024-23280336
E-mail:cyclonechen@126.com
http://www.lnkj.com.cn